History and perspectives of cardiology

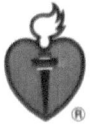 *This publication has been made possible through a grant from the Dutch Heart Foundation*

History and perspectives of cardiology

Catheterization, angiography, surgery and concepts of circular control

Edited by
H. A. SNELLEN, A. J. DUNNING and A. C. ARNTZENIUS

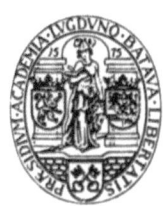

LEIDEN UNIVERSITY PRESS   THE HAGUE/BOSTON/LONDON

Distributors:

for the United States and Canada

Kluwer Boston, Inc.
190 Old Derby Street
Hingham, MA 02043
USA

for all other countries

Kluwer Academic Publishers Group
Distribution Center
P.O. Box 322
3300 AH Dordrecht
The Netherlands

This volume is listed in the Library of Congress Cataloging in Publication Data   CIP

Main entry under title:

History and perspectives of cardiology.

   Proceedings of the Einthoven meeting held at
Leiden University, Nov. 1-3, 1979.
   1. Cardiology--History--Congresses. I. Snellen,
H. A. II. Dunning, A. J. III. Arntzenius,
Alexander C. [DNLM: 1. Cardiology--Congresses.
2. Cardiology--History--Congresses. WG 11.1 H673
1979]
RC666.5.H57   616.1'2'009   81-12386
                                         AACR2

ISBN-13: 978-94-009-8623-7   e-ISBN-13: 978-94-009-8621-3
DOI: 10.1007/978-94-009-8621-3

Preface

The following presents the proceedings of the Einthoven meeting in Leiden, 1–2 November 1979. This meeting aimed at reviewing the historical development of a few selected cardiological topics as a continuous process. Essentially this means reviewing three phases: the early history, the recent past, and the present with an outlook to the future. Mainly because of the chosen fields – clearly our choice of heart catheterization, angiocardiography, and cardiac surgery was not accidental – the emphasis was on recent history, of which its pioneers and their contemporaries can still testify. The opportunity for the older generation to meet again, and for the younger to hear pioneers tell about their work and to listen to experts recreating the past as the forerunner of the present, was a unique and stimulating occasion enjoyed by old and young alike.

With great regret it was announced that Dr. Werner Forssmann, who had promised to attend the meeting and was looking forward to it, had died unexpectedly a few months ago. Instead of his personal contribution to the history of the pioneering age, a short tribute to his memory was paid by Dr. Loogen, professor of cardiology in Düsseldorf, and by Sir John McMichael, who showed part of an old movie on heart catheterization, in which Dr. Forssmann explained his part in this development.

In his welcoming address, Dr. Tammeling, the Dean of the Leiden Medical School, made clear that the university deeply appreciated the privilege of receiving this distinguished gathering. He referred to the tradition of experimental medicine in Leiden during the 17th century, leading to an early recognition of Harvey's work, which constituted the foundation of both physiology and cardiology. On the other hand, it is significant that the present meeting was dedicated to Einthoven, pioneer of cardiology and a lifelong member of Leiden University, whose memory for the last 25 years has been honored by a biennial Einthoven Lecture, given by today's pioneers in studying and combating heart disease. This time the Einthoven Lecture has been included in the program of the meeting and concerns a vital point of the circulation: its regulation.

Plans for subsequent meetings of the same type were discussed on the second day and are mentioned on page 79.

During the preparation of this volume, we learned that Lord Brock has passed away (September 1980). It is a great privilege to include his paper as a memory of this outstanding pioneer of cardiac surgery.

Contents

Contributors

Abrams, Herbert L.	*Department of Radiology, Harvard Medical School, Boston, Massachusetts, USA*
Arntzenius, A.C.	*Leiden University Hospital, Leiden, The Netherlands*
Bigelow, William G.	*Toronto General Hospital, Toronto, Canada*
Bing, Richard J.	*School of Medicine, University of Southern California, Los Angeles, California, USA*
Bost, Jack	*Ecole Nationale Vétérinaire de Lyon, Lyon, France*
Brock, Lord	*Deceased in September 1980*
Brom, A.G.	*Department of Thoracic Surgery, Leiden University Hospital, Leiden, The Netherlands*
Burch, George E.	*Department of Medicine, Tulane University School of Medicine, New Orleans, Louisiana, USA*
Castellanos, Agustin W.	*Coral Gables, Florida, USA*
Cournand, André F.	*College of Physicians and Surgeons, Columbia University, New York, New York, USA*
Crafoord, Clarence	*Karolinska Sjukhuset, Stockholm, Sweden*
Denolin, H.	*Hôpital St. Pierre, Brussels, Belgium*
Dexter, Lewis	*Peter Bent Brigham Hospital, Boston, Massachusetts USA*
Dunning, Arend J.	*Department of Internal Medicine, Binnengasthuis, University of Amsterdam, Amsterdam, The Netherlands*
Effler, Donald B.	*St. Joseph's Hospital Health Center, Syracuse, New York, USA*
Engelse, Willem A.H.	*Thorax Center, Erasmus University, Rotterdam, The Netherlands*
Guyton, Arthur C.	*Department of Physiology and Biophysics, University of Mississippi Medical Center, Jackson, Mississippi, USA*
Hoare, Mary Rose	*Thorax Center, Erasmus University, Rotterdam, The Netherlands*
Hugenholtz, Paul G.	*Thorax Center, Erasmus University, Rotterdam, The Netherlands*
Jönsson, Gunnar	*Stockholm, Sweden*
Loogen, Franz	*Department of Cardiology, University Hospital, Düsseldorf, FRG*
Maurice, Pierre	*Clinique Cardiologique, Hôpital Broussais, Paris, France*

McMichael, Sir John	*London, UK*
Reiber, Hans	*Thorax Center, Erasmus University, Rotterdam, The Netherlands*
Rullière, Roger	*Chaire Française d'Histoire de la Médecine et de la Chirurgie, Paris, France*
Sayers, Bruce McA.	*Imperial College of Science and Technology, Engineering in Medicine Laboratory, London, UK*
Schoot, Jan B. van der	*Department of Nuclear Medicine, Wilhelmina Gasthuis, University of Amsterdam, Amsterdam, The Netherlands*
Senning, Åke	*Chirurgische Universitätsklinik A, Zürich, Switzerland*
Simoons, Maarten L.	*Thorax Center, Erasmus University, Rotterdam, The Netherlands*
Snellen, Herman A.	*Oegstgeest, The Netherlands*
Mason Sones, F.	*Cleveland Clinic, Cleveland, Ohio, USA*
Sonolet, Jacqueline	*Musée d'Histoire de la Médecine, Paris, France*
Steinberg, Israel	*Abingdon, Virginia, USA*
Swan, Henry	*Lakewood, Colorado, USA*
Swan Peng Lie	*Thorax Center, Erasmus University, Rotterdam, The Netherlands*
Tammeling, G. J.	*Department of Physiology, Leiden University, Leiden, The Netherlands*
Taussig, Helen B.	*Kennett Square, Pennsylvania, USA*
Zeelenberg, Cees	*Thorax Center, Erasmus University, Rotterdam, The Netherlands*

PART ONE

History of heart catheterization and angiocardiography

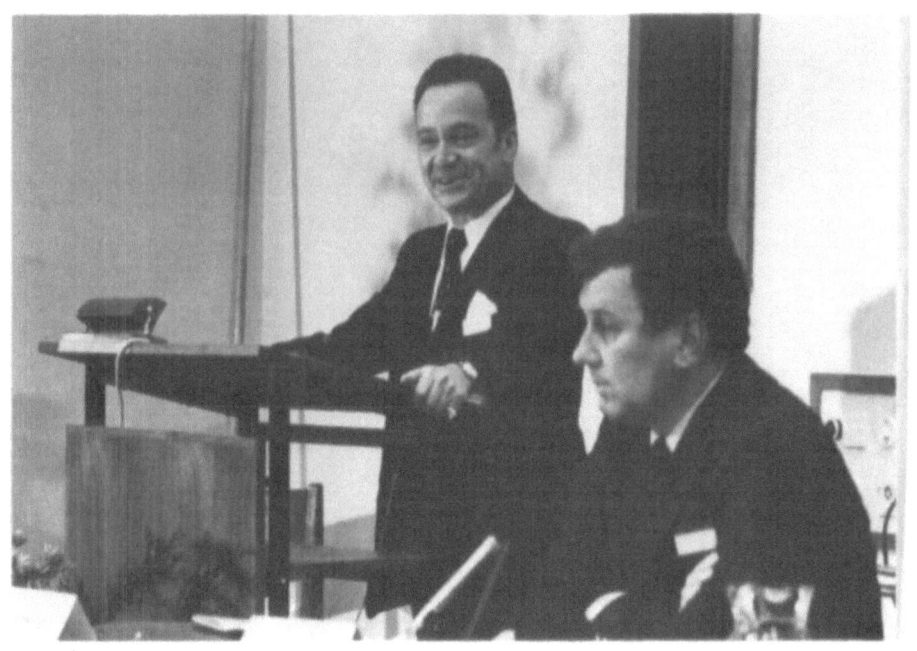

Dr. R. Rullière (left) and Dr. A.J. Dunning, chairman of the session.

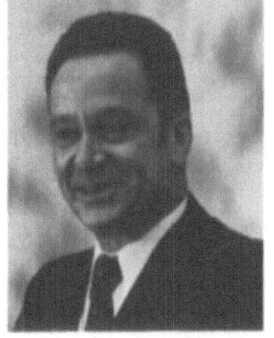

R. RULLIÈRE / J. SONOLET

Roger Rullière is titular professor of medical history in Paris, as well as being an active cardiologist at a Paris teaching hospital. He has made several contributions to electrocardiography, particularly its clinical use, and has written several papers on the history of cardiology, especially on cardiology in the 19th century.

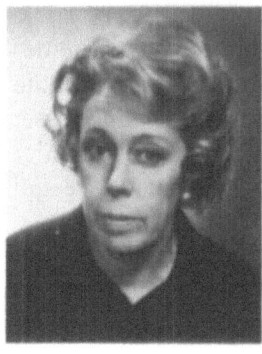

Miss Jacqueline Sonolet, who prepared the historical note on Marey with Dr. Rullière, has been responsible for a considerable time for promoting interest in the history of medicine in her double function: curator of the Museum of History of Medicine in Paris as well as curator of the Museum of Claude Bernard in St. Julien (Beaujolais).

Claude Bernard et le cathétérisme cardiaque

Claude Bernard est un précurseur essentiel dans l'histoire du cathétérisme expérimental chez les animaux. On en retrouve la trace dans ses Cahiers d'expériences ainsi que dans ses Leçons sur les liquides de l'organisme, la chaleur animale et la physiologie opératoire.

Lavoisier avait, en 1785, situé la combustion au niveau des poumons. Il était donc sous-entendu que, dans cette hypothèse, le sang artériel devait être plus chaud que le sang veineux.

Plusieurs auteurs semblaient l'avoir confirmé, tels Haller (1760), Crawford (1778), Saissy (1808), Davy (1815), Krimer (1823), Scudamore (1826), Becquerel et Brechet (1837), et Nasse (1843).

En revanche, Collard de Martigny et Malgaigne en 1832, Berger en 1833 et Magnus en 1842 (ce dernier par l'étude des gaz du sang) affirmaient que le processus de combustion se produisait au niveau des tissus périphériques et que le sang veineux devait être plus chaud que le sang artériel. C'est aux mêmes conclusions que devaient aboutir Hering en 1850 et Liebig en 1854.

Il faut remarquer toutefois que la plupart des protocoles d'expériences étaient contestables et c'est pourquoi Claude Bernard envisagea d'aller étudier la température du sang dans les cavités cardiaques et chez l'animal vivant, au

3

lieu de se contenter de le faire au niveau des vaisseaux, ou chez l'animal mort, ou chez l'animal thoracotomisé.

Ses premières expériences furent effectuées en 1844 avec François Magendie, sur des chevaux morveux. Sa seconde expérience fut faite chez le chien, le 22 novembre 1848. Mais la plupart des expériences eurent lieu après 1850. Une première série porte, de mai 1853 à juillet 1856, sur 10 chiens. Une deuxième série d'expériences porte sur 14 moutons, les 9 et 16 juin 1853 et le 9 mars 1854.

La voie d'abord pour le cathétérisme droit est, dans l'immense majorité des expériences, la voie jugulaire. Claude Bernard insiste sur son extrême facilité et montre que si l'on peut aller dans le ventricule droit, on peut aussi pousser la sonde dans la veine cave inférieure. Mais, il dit aussi qu'on peut pénétrer par les veines crurales et conseille surtout la veine crurale gauche, ce qui facilite le passage au niveau de l'abouchement des veines sus-hépatiques.

La voie d'abord pour le cathétérisme gauche est dans l'immense majorité des cas la voie carotidienne. Claude Bernard souligne la difficulté du franchissement des valvules sigmoïdes d'autant, dit-il, que ces sigmoïdes ne sont jamais complètement ouvertes au cours de la systole. Il lui semble plus simple de passer par la carotide gauche à condition d'avoir couché le chien du côté droit. Il souligne le risque de perforer les sigmoïdes. Claude Bernard montre que l'on peut aussi atteindre le ventricule gauche en partant de l'artère crurale, surtout si l'on s'adresse à l'artère crurale droite: c'est donc un précurseur du cathétérisme rétrograde des cavités gauches.

Les sondes employées par Claude Bernard sont soit des thermomètres, soit des systèmes «thermométriques». En 1844, il dit avoir utilisé un «long thermomètre». En 1856, il a utilisé un thermomètre à alcool. Mais, la plupart de ses expériences ont été faites, soit avec une sonde thermo-électrique notamment en ce qui concerne les chiens, soit avec le thermomètre métastatique à mercure de Walferdin en ce qui concerne les moutons. Pour ce qui est des sondes thermo-électriques, il dit lui-même qu'il utilisait «deux sondes souples de gomme élastique» qui contiennent chacune un fil de cuivre et un fil de fer, lesquels sont reliés à un galvanomètre qui indique des différences de température. Entre parenthèses, Claude Bernard, dans ces conditions, effectue un cathétérisme simultanément droit et gauche. En revanche, le thermomètre métastatique est plongé alternativement jusqu'au ventricule droit, puis jusqu'au ventricule gauche, ou inversement.

L'ensemble de ces expériences démontre à Claude Bernard que, dans le cœur, le sang veineux est plus chaud, en moyenne de 1 ou 2/10e de degré, que le sang artériel et que, par conséquent, le sang se refroidit en traversant les poumons. Après 1856, Claude Bernard dresse une véritable cartographie de la chaleur animale et des températures des sangs afférent et efférent de divers organes montrant que le sang veineux est habituellement nettement plus chaud que le sang artériel, apportant ainsi des preuves définitives que les phénomènes de combustion sont bien viscéraux et périphériques.

En conclusion, les cathétérismes cardiaques de Claude Bernard sont plus l'œuvre d'un physicien et d'un biologiste que celle d'un cardiologue. Ses préoccupations ne sont nullement hémodynamiques, contrairement à celles de Chauveau et de Marey, et Claude Bernard dit lui-même: «tout le monde connaît les belles expériences par lesquelles Chauveau et Marey ont pu déterminer, en introduisant des sondes dans les oreillettes et les ventricules, les pressions que développent ces cavités lors de leurs contractions et établir avec précision le synchronisme de ces contractions». Mais, ce n'était pas là le problème de Claude Bernard.

BIBLIOGRAPHIE

Cahiers d'expériences de Claude Bernard. Collège de France.
Leçons sur les propriétés physiologiques et les altérations pathologiques des liquides de l'organisme, 5ᵉ leçon. Paris: Baillière éditeur, 1859.
Leçons sur la chaleur animale (leçons de 1871–1872), 3ᵉ, 5ᵉ et 6ᵉ leçons. Paris: Baillière éditeur, 1876.
Leçons de physiologie opératoire. 12ᵉ leçon. Paris: Baillière éditeur, 1879.

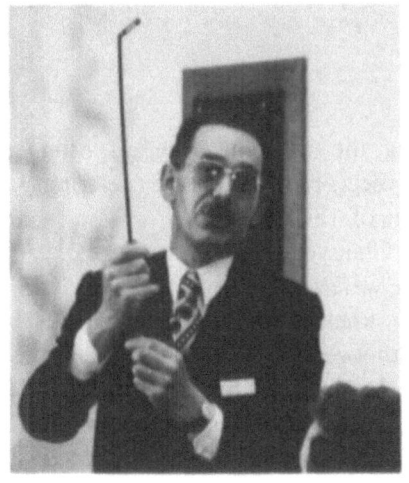

JACK BOST

Jack Bost showing the Chauveau and Marey catheter. Dr. Bost, born in 1925, is a veterinarian and has been chairman of the Department of Physiology and Pharmacology of the Veterinary School of Lyon since 1959. His chief interests lie in the physiology of the circulation and in the history of biological sciences.

Chauveau and Marey's accomplishment: the first intracardiac pressure records

After so many controversial experiments and discussions, the mechanical functions of the heart seemed to be definitely settled in 1855. In that year, a 28-year-old assistant at the Department of Anatomy of the Veterinary School of Lyon, J.B.A. Chauveau, had performed a thorough study on the cardiac cycle in open-chest horses. While working with the cardiologist Faivre, Chauveau had reinforced most of Harvey's old statements. However, Beau, a physician from Paris, still refused to acknowledge that the apex beat was a phenomenon of ventricular systole. According to him, it was obviously impossible for the apex to hit the chest at the time when ventricular volume suddenly decreased in size. It was evident, so he thought, that the impulse of the apex had to arise from the increased ventricular volume which results from its filling due to atrial contraction. In April 1861, Beau enforced his theory with a public demonstration (on frog, tortoise, and eel hearts) at the French Société de Biologie.

In 1902, addressing Marey, Chauveau recalled that he had met Marey by chance at the Veterinary School of Alfort when the latter, a former student of Beau, had already prepared an experiment for demonstrating his master's theory. The demonstration failed and the two physiologists decided to associate. As a gift to this association, Chauveau brought his vast knowledge of equine anatomy and his experience in heart physiology. Marey, for his part, was the bright young French leader of the new registration techniques first introduced by Carl Ludwig in 1847. He had already given proofs of his remarkable ingenuity in the field of improving or devising physiological apparatus, namely the sphygmograph. Working together was not easy: Chauveau lived in Lyon, whereas Marey lived in Paris. Moreover, Chauveau recalls that he himself worked only during the morning whereas Marey worked by night. However, they managed to meet, probably at the Veterinary School of Alfort during the summer vacation of 1861.

Turning now to the technical details of Chauveau and Marey's experiments, there is no doubt that both of them were well informed on Claude Bernard's achievements. In consequence, they knew of the feasibility to push catheters into the heart of a standing unanesthetized horse, through the large vessels of the neck. As early as in 1858, Marey had made unsuccessful attempts at intracardiac pressure recording. He had used water transmission with a lead tube which resulted in considerable damping of pressure waves. Success was brought on by the welcome contribution of a forgotten French physiologist, Charles Buisson. In March 1861, Buisson presented a new sphygmograph at the Société de Biologie. The apparatus was made of two small regular glass funnels covered by rubber membrane and connected by rubber tubing. One of them was used as a transducer (pressed against an artery), the other one (fitted with a light straw lever) as a recorder. This was to become the famous and long-lived Marey's tambour. There is no doubt that the idea of air transmission was a revelation for Chauveau and Marey, who immediately started to devise their cardiac catheter. They probably worked in a hurry as they were able to publish the first ever made record of intracardiac pressures at the Académie des Sciences on 7 October 1861, only six months after Buisson's communication. What are the contents of this short note of three pages, including one figure? They had used a flexible double-lumen catheter fitted with two rubber ampullae. The catheter had been threaded into the jugular vein until the terminal ampulla reached the right ventricle. The distance between the two ampullae was such that the second one then stayed inside the right auricle. Yet another ampulla had been inserted between the chest wall and the heart in order to record the apex beat. Each ampulla was connected via rubber tubing to a tambour the lever of which wrote on blackened paper on the recording drum. The published record clearly shows that atrial systole is well finished by the time that the apex beat begins simultaneously with the onset of ventricular systole. In fact, registered evidence of Harvey's statements was brought forth for the first time.

But this is not the end of the story. Beau then made an accurate study of Chauveau's note and pointed toward a very serious defect of the record. During atrial systole, the ventricular pressure line stayed perfectly flat. So, he asked, where does the blood go which is expelled by the auricle, if it does not go into the ventricle? This criticism urged Chauveau and Marey to improve the sensitivity and accuracy of their experimental device. On 6 January 1862, at the Académie des Sciences, they issued a second record on which a conspicuous rise of ventricular pressure can be seen to occur at the time of atrial systole.

(The left ventricular pressure curve does not appear on this record, neither does it on a third record presented to the Académie de Médecine in 1863. However, simultaneous catheterization of right and left ventricles, with measurement of actual intracardiac pressures, had been achieved during the year 1862, as was mentioned by Claude Bernard in a special report [on candidates for the yearly Prize of Physiology] read by him to the Académie des Sciences on 22 December 1862.)

At that time, scientific Academies still kept to the straightest concept of their duty as warrants of truth and, as the registration technique still met with a great deal of skepticism, the Academies often requested the authors to repeat their experiments publicly, under control of an elected commission. When asked to do this, Chauveau and Marey passed this trial successfully during 1862, under the supervision of Milne-Edwards, chairman of the commission. However, Beau was such a stubborn character that he resumed his criticism. He went so far in his unfairness that he suspected Chauveau and Marey to have purposely tampered with their device in order to get the required record! He was such a controversialist that he brought the discussion to the Académie de Médecine of Paris in 1864 where it lasted for three months, during 11 out of the 14 meetings of that period. The proceedings of these sessions amount to 245 printed pages. When, at last, the discussion was closed, Beau said 'je crois inutile de répondre: je n'ai rien à ajouter ni à retrancher. Je remercie seulement l'Académie de l'attention qu'elle a bien voulu me prêter'.

In conclusion, Chauveau and Marey's intracardiac records, the cornerstone of modern cardiology, seem to result from a coincidence of several scientific, technical, and human factors:

— first of all, the fortuitous association of two exceptionally skilled physiologists;
— secondly, the unexpected invention of a very simple air transmission sphygmograph by Buisson; and
— thirdly, the incentive of a hot controversy and the stubbornness of Beau.

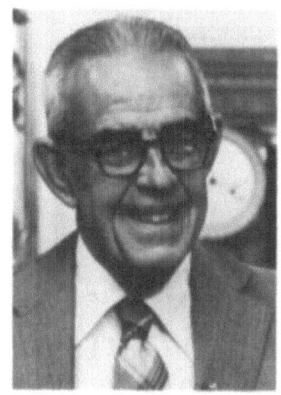

LEWIS DEXTER

Lewis Dexter, born in 1910, was associated with the Peter Bent Brigham Hospital and Harvard Medical School (Boston, USA) from 1941 till 1976, lastly as professor of medicine. His fundamental contribution was made during the second world war when Dr. Dexter and his team were the first to study the heart by right-sided catheterization.

A brief history of the clinical application of cardiac catheterization, 1929–1979

It is a pleasure as well as a privilege for me to participate in this meeting. I thank you from the bottom of all four chambers of my heart. This meeting is to honor one of the greatest contributors to cardiology – Willem Einthoven of Leiden. I doubt if he realized that, 76 years later, the medical profession would still be using the electrocardiogram as a routine test, as well as studying and actively investigating the secrets of its recordings. I cannot think of any other method, with the possible exception of the X-ray, that has had such long-lasting usage, utility, and intellectual challenge. Not only that: the string-galvanometer was the perfect instrument, yielding tracings far superior to almost anything we have today. I must correct one error of the program. I was not the first to perform right-heart catheterization; the credit goes to the late Drs. Forssmann and Richards, and to Dr. Cournand.

I have been asked to give a brief history of the clinical application of the technique of cardiac catheterization. As you all know, it is a technique whereby a catheter is introduced into the vascular system and then, by sampling of blood, injecting of substances or measuring pressures from one or another part of the venous or arterial system or heart itself, a wide variety of physiologic, metabolic, and anatomic studies become possible.

For convenience, the history of the catheter can be divided into decades as follows:

Historical decades of the cardiac catheter

1929–39 Forssmann
1940–49 Richards and Cournand; early beginnings

1950-59 Epidemic spread (open-heart surgery)
1960-69 Continuation (CABG surgery)
1970-79 Waning of its use (noninvasive techniques)
1980-   The future

1929-1939

Although one or two others preceded Werner Forssmann, it all really began
with him in 1929, when he inserted a catheter into the vein of his own
forearm, guided it fluoroscopically into his right atrium, took an X-ray picture
of the catheter in this position, and reported no discomfort from the procedure. He was allegedly severely criticized for doing such a foolish thing, but
was subsequently given the world's greatest medical award – the Nobel
Prize – for his endeavor. It was used only sporadically during the 1930s by a
small number of people as, for example, Radner of Sweden.

1940-1949

I hope you realize that it is impossible for me to give more than a bird's-eye
view of the development of cardiac catheterization in the 1940s. However, let
me give you the names of those using the catheter in that decade. Richards
and Cournand, who also received the Nobel Prize, and their colleagues were
the only ones using the catheter in 1941-43. In 1944, there were two
more – Bradley in Boston and McMichael in London; in 1945, Stead, Warren,
and several colleagues in Atlanta, and Maurice and the late Professor Lenègre
in Paris, and myself in Boston; in 1946, Geiger in New Haven; in 1947, Bing
and Van Dam in Baltimore, Dorbrecker and Chavez in Mexico, Werkö in
Stockholm and Johnson in Montreal; in 1948, Laubry and Denolin in Paris,
Hansen and Lagerlöf in Copenhagen, Earl Wood at the Mayo Clinic, Soulié in
Paris, and Van Lingen in Johannesburg. In 1949, the number of catheterizers
more than doubled.

In 1940, knowledge of cardiac and circulatory physiology in animals was
quite extensive, thanks to Starling, Wiggers and others, but practically nothing was known about it in normal and in diseased man. The 1940s was an
exploratory period wherein methodology was excellent for measuring O_2 and
CO_2 in air and blood (i.e. for calculating cardiac output by the direct Fick
method), but until the late 1940s, pressure recorders were either optical or
mechanical and of variable quality.

Many of the workers in the 1940s measured the cardiac output in normals,
in a wide range of diseases, and during exercise. Flows were measured

through organs such as the liver, kidney, brain, and heart. Pressures were measured and analyzed from the right atrium, right ventricle, pulmonary artery, and pulmonary artery wedge positions in health and disease.

Disease entities were studied in some detail: shock, heart failure, pulmonary disease, pregnancy, congenital heart diseases, and mitral stenosis. Use of the catheter for precise diagnosis of surgically correctable heart disease was beginning to get under way. By the late 1940s, the surgically correctable lesions were patent ductus arteriosus, tetralogy of Fallot, coarctation of aorta, pulmonic stenosis, and mitral stenosis.

1950–1959

This decade was characterized by such progress in cardiology as the world had never seen before. Cardiac surgery and cardiac catheterization began to enjoy a symbiotic relationship. I shall make no attempt to name individuals responsible for the many advances because the list is endless.

1) Catheterization of not only the right but also the left side of the heart became routine.
2) Great expansion of cardiac surgery, particularly stimulated by the development of the extracorporeal pump in 1955, allowed for the first time intracardiac surgery under direct vision.
3) A correspondingly large number of catheterization laboratories appeared.
4) Investigation was carried out in depth of the physiology of all the surgically correctable as well as noncorrectable heart diseases – congenital heart diseases, mitral stenosis, constrictive pericarditis, cardiomyopathies, and myocardial failure.
5) Many new diagnostic methods were developed – special types of catheter, dye indicators, radioactive-isotopic indicators, hydrogen and oxygen electrodes, catheter tip manometers, and flow meters, together with suitable electronic recording instruments of high fidelity.
6) Physiology was correlated with anatomy, clinical manifestations, electrocardiogram, and radiology of a whole host of heart diseases.

As I look back at it, this was probably the most exciting period of all, the preceding decade having had so many puzzling and frustrating methodological and interpretative aspects, the succeeding decades having fewer unstudied diseases.

1960–1969

This decade was characterized by two great surgical advances – valve replacement and coronary artery bypass surgery.

It had been shown by Hufnagel in 1954 that implanted prosthetic valves were durable for years. Their implantation in 1960 in the root of the aorta proximal to the orifices of the coronary artery heralded a new era in valve surgery. Stenosis and, for the first time, regurgitation of all valves could now be corrected. This led to a redoubling of effort of assessment before as well as after surgery by cardiac catheterization. Many studies of myocardial function, as opposed to valve function, were now being undertaken by more and more sophisticated techniques involving especially the examination of isovolumic systole.

Many studies of the coronary circulation in man had been made initially by Bing beginning in the 1940s and later by him and others. Many had obtained good coronary arteriograms in the 1940s and 1950s, but the selective procedure of Sones in 1960 replaced all the others and is now the accepted method. Coronary surgery had been undertaken by Beck, Vineberg, Harken and others, but the method of coronary artery bypass grafting by Favaloro in 1965 resulted in the widespread implementation of this surgery in the United States and, to a lesser extent, elsewhere. It led, however, to an enormous amount of study of coronary artery disease – anatomy, myocardial contractility and contraction patterns, electrocardiography, exercise testing, and so forth. Central to all these studies was the use of the catheter for selective coronary arteriography, left ventricular angiography to determine the contraction pattern and chamber volume, the left ventricular systolic and diastolic pressures and output, the coronary blood flow, pressures, and resistances, and coronary sinus sampling for metabolic studies.

1970–1979

This decade saw the introduction of an impressive array of noninvasive methods which replaced many uses of the catheter, particularly in congenital heart disease, heart failure, pericardial disease, and to a certain extent in valvular heart disease.

1) Systolic time intervals yielded information on left ventricular function and contractility.
2) Both M-mode and two-dimensional echocardiography gave spectacular visualization of cardiac chambers, valves, septa, wall motion, wall thickness, great vessels, septal defects, and pericardial space from which con-

tractility, chamber volumes, ejection fraction, cardiac output, location and direction of shunts, IHSS, and mitral valve prolapse could be visualized or measured.
3) The technology of radionuclide angiography developed to such an extent in this decade as to allow the calculation of ejection fraction, the estimation of chamber volumes and wall motion as well as measurement of cardiac output and localization, quantification and direction of intracardiac shunts.

These three noninvasive methods have to a great extent reduced the use of the cardiac catheter.

RÉSUMÉ AND FUTURE (1980–)

The cardiac catheter has elucidated cardiac behavior in health and disease as no previous or current method could have done. It came into being at about the same time as cardiac surgery. Without the catheter, cardiac surgery could not have advanced as it did. Without cardiac surgery, the catheter would have had limited usage. But it was far more than a diagnostic tool. It revealed many facets of cardiac, pulmonary, hepatic, renal, and cerebral physiology and metabolism by its ability to make possible the measurement of pressure and flow and of substances in arterial inflow and venous outflow. For example, the differences in knowledge of congenital heart disease now as compared with 1945 when Maude Abbott's atlas and James Brown's little book on congenital heart disease were my 'bibles' is impressive because, for the first time, it was possible to make a precise diagnosis antemortem, and this was entirely due to catheterization. This applies as well to many other forms of heart disease such as mitral regurgitation, which was considered to be unimportant in the 1940s and is now the commonest valvular disease.

But what of the future of the catheter. Has it had its use and will it now fade away? The answer to this is no for the foreseeable future. The heart is a pressure-flow organ. Although flows can be measured noninvasively, pressures cannot, at least for the forseeable future. Systolic pressures in the left ventricle can be deduced from the arterial systolic pressure in the absence of aortic stenosis, but precise measurement, including that in diastole, requires direct measurement for studies of systole, diastolic relaxation, and myocardial contractility.

In aortic stenosis and mitral stenosis, left ventricular pressure must be recorded in order to measure the pressure gradient across the valve, which, in turn, is necessary for the calculation of the severity of the stenosis. The pressure gradient across the lung must be recorded for the calculation of pulmonary vascular resistance which, when sufficiently elevated, negates the effectiveness of cardiac surgery in those with congenital heart disease.

The catheter will continue to be of value in the study of metabolic activity of all organs. It has already been shown to be of great value in relieving atherosclerotic obstructions by transluminal balloon dilatation in peripheral vascular disease and in certain cases of coronary artery disease. This technique is still in its infancy and with more experience may have much more widespread application. Its continued use for selective angiography of all parts of the body seems assured. Until atherosclerosis is controlled medically, coronary arteriography will be a prerequisite to coronary artery bypass grafting.

Cardiac catheterization has thus had a glorious history in increasing our knowledge of heart disease. Although its use is waning, it promises to continue to be used as a diagnostic and investigative technique and as the gold standard with which other methods are compared.

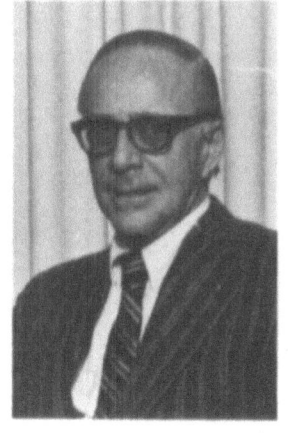

HERBERT L. ABRAMS

Herbert L. Abrams, born in 1920, was professor of radiology at the Stanford University School of Medicine till 1967 and thereafter held the same post at Harvard Medical School, where he is the chief radiologist at Peter Bent Brigham Hospital in Boston. His main interest over the years has been angiography of heart and vessels, both experimentally and clinically. He is the editor of the standard textbook of angiography and has contributed to numerous innovations in cineangiography, selective catheterization, renovascular hypertension, and computed tomography.

The development of angiocardiography

Historically, the origins of a new and important diagnostic technique are often totally unrelated to its most important application. This is as true of angiocardiography as of the entire field of roentgenology.

On 8 November 1895, Roentgen, while experimenting with the Hittorf-Crookes tube, observed a bright fluorescence of barium platinocyanide crystals. He assumed initially that the fluorescence might be caused by cathode (beta) rays. Using a fluorescent screen, he removed it beyond the range of cathode rays; when the fluorescence persisted he became aware that the effect was produced by a new kind of rays. Not long afterward, he replaced the screen with a recording photographic plate. One of the dramatic results of this experiment was a picture of his wife's hand. On 28 December 1895, after eight weeks of intensive investigation, he delivered the manuscript reporting his discovery of X-rays[1] (Fig. 1). His two classic papers of March 1896 and May 1897 completed the recording of many fundamental observations, to which little was added for many years.

By early January 1896, word of Roentgen's discovery and its import had spread around the world[2]. Almost immediately, the possibilities of applying the new 'photography' to traumatic lesions of bone fired the imagination and, within a month, X-rays of fractures had been obtained and published. Early in the year, Edison and many others began intensive work on the fluoroscope. By the end of March 1896, Becher had outlined the stomach and intestines of a sacrificed guinea pig with lead subacetate and mentioned the idea of delineating fistulas in this way[3]. In the fall of 1896, Walter B. Cannon, a physiologist who was interested in the motor activities of the

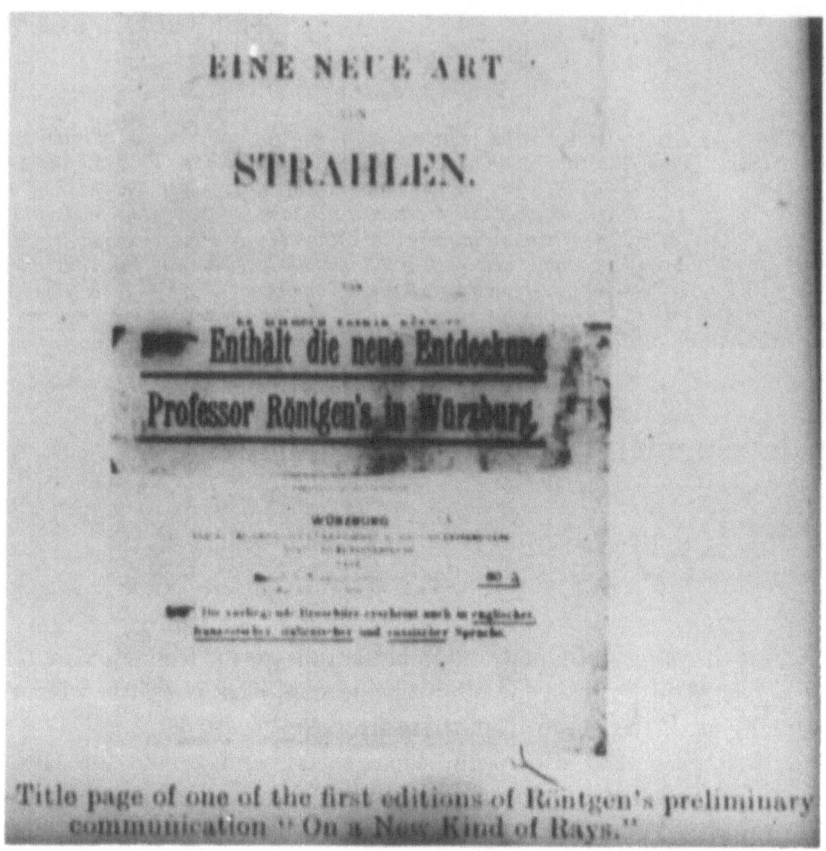

Fig. 1. On 28 December 1895, Roentgen reports his discovery of X-rays.

stomach, undertook a study in cats suggested to him by H. P. Bowditch of Boston. Mixing bismuth subnitrate with the food, he subsequently described in detail the nature and site of peristaltic activity as he saw it on the fluoroscopic screen [4].

Visualization of the blood vessels in man was achieved early in the year. In January 1896, during the month after the announcement of Roentgen's discovery, Haschek and Lindenthal injected Teichman's mixture into the blood vessels of an amputated hand [5] (Figs. 2 and 3). A photograph of their original roentgenogram was published in a January issue of the *Wiener Klinische Wochenschrift* and showed clearly the potential of the method for visualizing the vascular bed. A volume by Morton written in 1896 is of interest in this regard [6]. His remarks about contrast studies are intriguing:

In teaching the anatomy of the blood vessels, the X-ray opens out a new and feasible method. The arteries and veins of dead bodies may be injected with a substance opaque to the X-ray and thus, their distribution may be more accurately followed than by any possible dissection. The feasibility of this method applies equally well to the study of the structures and organs of the dead body. To a certain extent, therefore, X-ray photography may replace both dissection and vivisection, and in the living body, the location and size of a hollow organ may be ascertained.

At the time that Voelcker and von Lichtenberg introduced retrograde myelography to the field of urographic diagnosis in 1906 [7], a number of medical schools had organized departments of roentgenology.

In 1920, an X-ray atlas devoted only to the 'Systematic Arteries of the Body' was published in England [8]. In it were roentgenographic reproductions which showed the blood vessels in cadavers with great clarity.

Meanwhile Franck and Alwens, in 1910, introduced a suspension of bismuth and oil into the heart of dogs and rabbits directly through the large veins [9]. They were able to observe the passage of the oily droplets from the heart into the lungs. The work of Sicard and Forestier, twelve years later, represented the next major advance. They had employed Lipiodol to study first the bronchial tree and then the spinal subarachnoid space in 1922. A year later, they decided to try the oil in the cardiovascular system [10]. Working with dogs, they slowly injected 5 cc of Lipiodol into the femoral vein and, with the aid of fluoroscopy, watched the droplets move with

---

Aus dem physik.-chem. Institute des Prof. Franz Exner.

Ein Beitrag zur praktischen Verwerthung der Photographie nach Röntgen.

Von E. Haschek und Dr. O. Th. Lindenthal.

Das grosse Interesse, welches die gesammte gebildete Welt der neuen Entdeckung Professor Röntgen's entgegenbringt, veranlasste uns zu einigen Versuchen, welche zeigen sollten, in welcher Weise die Medicin sich die neuen Strahlen zu Nutzen machen könnte.

Als Lichtquelle diente eine ballonförmige Crooker'sche Röhre, die durch einen kräftigen Ruhmkorff'schen Inductionsapparat zur Phosphorescenz gebracht wurde; sie war derart befestigt, dass die Kathode ungefähr 20 cm vertical über die, für gewöhnliches Licht völlig undurchdringliche photographische Cassette zu liegen kam. Die zu untersuchenden Objecte wurden direct auf die geschlossene Cassette aufgelegt und ungefähr eine Stunde lang den Röntgen'schen X-Strahlen ausgesetzt.

Nachdem der Röntgen'sche Originalversuch; die Knochen innerhalb der lebenden Hand zur Anschauung zu bringen,

---

Fig. 2. In January 1896, Haschek and Lindenthal describe the potential of Roentgen's discovery for medicine.

19

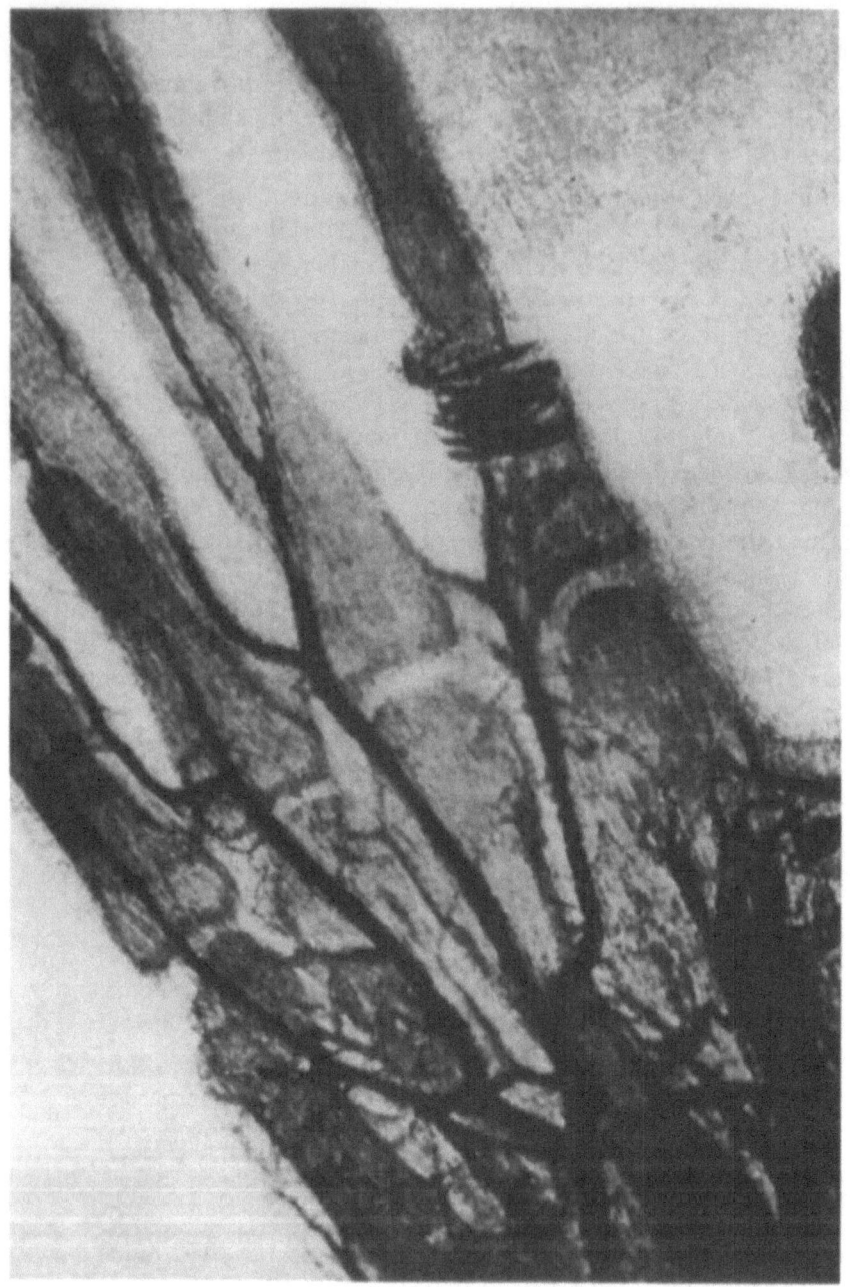

Fig. 3. Blood vessels of an amputated hand visualized by Haschek and Lindenthal (1896).

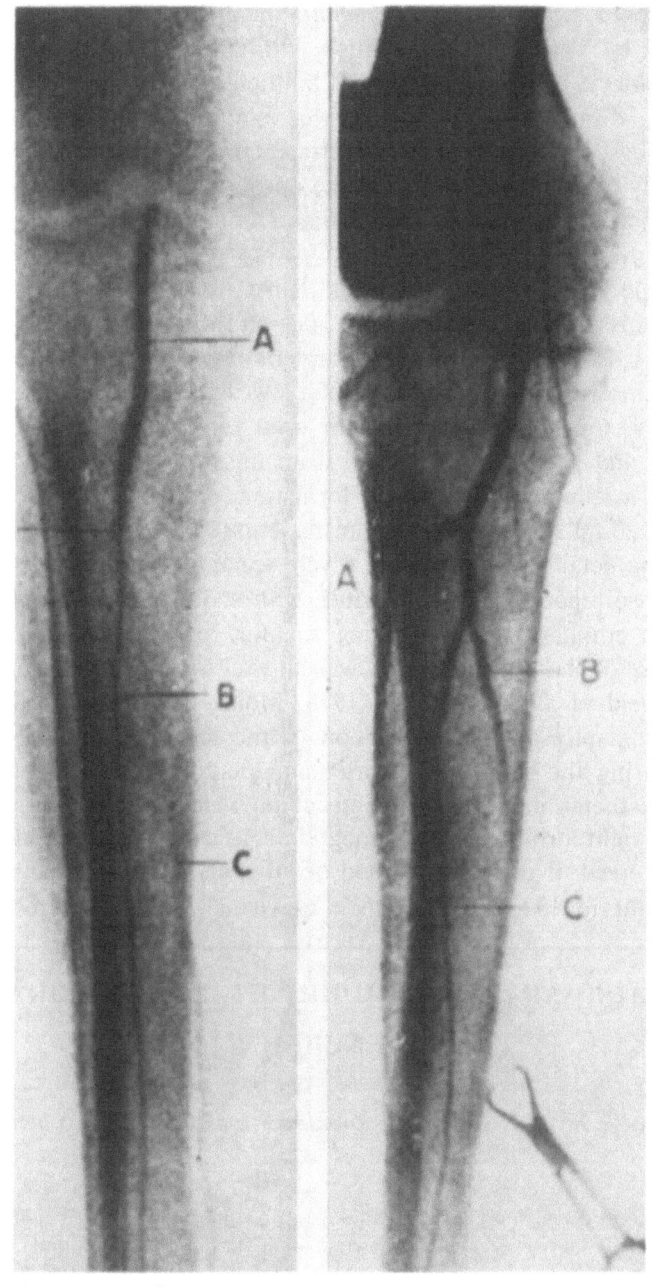

Fig. 4. Intraarterial injection of sodium iodide as a means of demonstrating the vessels of the lower extremity in man (1924, Brooks).

increasing speed from the iliac vein into the heart. The Lipiodol was then 'pulverized' by ventricular contraction, thrown with great speed into the pulmonary artery, and finally spread as multiple emboli into the small vessels of the lung, disappearing in ten to twelve minutes. Emboldened by their success in dogs, they repeated the experiment with human subjects, in whom they carefully observed the course of the opaque oil from the antecubital vein to the pulmonary capillaries. Their patients coughed as the oil reached the lungs but suffered no other ill effects.

In the same year, 1923, Berberich and Hirsch reported the first arteriograms and venograms obtained in man, with 20% strontium bromide [11]. One year later, in 1924, Brooks reported the intraarterial injection of sodium iodide as a means of demonstrating the vessels of the lower extremity in man [12] (Fig. 4). Subsequently, Carnett and Greenbaum used Lipiodol for arteriography, but its viscosity and globulation rendered it an unsatisfactory agent [13]. Saito et al., in order to eliminate the globule formation, emulsified Lipiodol and used as much as 20 ml for arteriography in patients [14]. Their studies were quite clear, and the detail satisfactory. No severe reactions were reported. Charbonnel and Massé reported their experience with sodium iodide in arteriography in 1929, but emphasized the irritating qualities of the agent [15].

The decade of the twenties, then, was an exciting developmental period for the entire field of angiography. In 1928, Moniz described the technique of carotid angiography and its application to the study of cerebral lesions [16] (Fig. 5). During the same year, Forssmann, having practiced on a cadaver, inserted a catheter into his own antecubital vein until he felt that it had reached the right atrium. A roentgenogram confirmed his supposition. Originally he conceived of this as a method of infusing therapeutic substances into the heart, but in 1931 he undertook to visualize the right heart and the

---

LA RADIO-ARTÉRIOGRAPHIE ET LA TOPOGRAPHIE
CRANIO-ENCÉPHALIQUE

Par EGAS MONIZ, ALMEIDA DIAS et ALMEIDA LIMA (Lisbonne).

.a radiographie est un précieux aide des travaux anatomiques et il nous semble q
nous donner des renseignements importants dans la détermination de la position d
s artères. Nous l'avons mise à profit dans l'étude de la circulation artérielle cérébrale
niner la distribution artérielle du crâne.
.orsque nous sommes arrivés à rendre visible le réseau artériel par des liquides op

---

Fig. 5. In 1928, Moniz describes the technique of carotid angiography.

pulmonary vessels with Uroselectan[17]. He succeeded in dogs but not in human subjects. Dos Santos, in 1929, showed that satisfactory opacification of the abdominal aorta and its branches could be obtained by using translumbar needle puncture and injection[18]. The Portuguese, pioneers in the field of angiography, also addressed themselves to the problem of showing the pulmonary vessels in disease. In 1931, using sodium iodide. Moniz and his colleagues devised the technique of 'angiopneumography,' as they called it, and described the appearance of the pulmonary vessels in a variety of conditions[19]. They were unable to visualize the cardiac chambers.

In 1929, Swick reported the use of an organic iodide, synthesized by Binz and Rath[20, 21], known as Selectan[22]. The discovery of an opaque organic iodide which was moderately well tolerated when administered intravenously was of immense importance to the field of angiography. Selectan was supplemented by Neoselectan (Iopax) and then by Uroselectan B (Neo-Iopax). Soon thereafter, Abrodil (Skiodan) was synthesized, to be replaced by Per-Abrodil (Diodrast).

By 1931, Skiodan had been employed in arteriography[23, 24] and venography[25, 26] with gratifying results, and within the next few years a number of studies of varicose veins were reported[27, 28]. The organic iodides, then, were introduced at a time when femoral, brachial, and carotid arteriography, venography, and translumbar aortography had all been accomplished, but were dependent in large measure on a relatively noxious agent, sodium iodide. Satisfactory opacification of the heart and great thoracic arteries had not yet been attained.

In 1933, Rousthöi, working with the experimental animal, described the opacification of the cardiac chambers and the aorta in an important paper called 'Über Angiokardiographie'[29]. During succeeding years a number of investigators[30–32] attempted to opacify the heart in man before Ameuille, in 1936, finally succeeded in doing so using the catheter method[33]. A year later the first practical method of angiocardiography was described[34].

As far back as 1931, Castellanos had undertaken the investigation of congenital cardiac anomalies by injecting sodium iodide intravenously and immediately thereafter obtaining a roentgenogram. This represented the first effort to apply the technique of intravenous injection of opaque material to the diagnosis of congenital heart disease. Castellanos felt, however, that sodium iodide was too toxic a material for satisfactory intravenous use in humans, and hence he discontinued his investigations until a more satisfactory substance was available. Meanwhile, he carefully explored the diagnostic implications of the technique on cadavers. Satisfied, at length, that Perabrodil (a trade name for Iodopyracet or Diodrast) combined adequate contrast with relatively slight toxicity, he tried it in humans.

Late in 1937, Castellanos, Pereiras, and Garcia reported the first successful roentgen contrast diagnosis of a number of congenital cardiac anomalies during life. This report constituted an astonishingly complete summary of a carefully conceived and well-executed investigation of the possibilities of 'angiocardiography,' the name they applied to this technique. Between September 1937 and July 1938, they published many papers in a number of journals, elaborating on the technique and summarizing the diagnostic criteria [34–40]. By July 1938, when Robb and Steinberg independently reported the successful opacification of the right and left cardiac chambers, Castellanos and his group had described the angiocardiographic appearance of many of the entities virtually as we know them today. They had published illustrations of atrial and ventricular septal defects, pulmonic stenosis, the tetralogy of Fallot, and transposition of the great vessels; had suggested and performed biplane studies; and had devised an automatic injection device which they described in some detail. Their initial contributions were extraordinarily impressive.

One gap in their method of investigating the heart in the living subject was that they were able to opacify adequately only the right heart chambers. Actually, this was sufficient for establishing the diagnosis in many congenital anomalies, since it demonstrated the transposed or 'overriding' aorta, pulmonic stenosis and, at times, defects in the cardiac septa. Another early limitation they encountered was that satisfactory visualization occurred inconsistently; it was most regularly obtained in children under the age of two years, was occasionally obtained in those two to six years old, and was rarely achieved in those over the age of six years [34]. By May of 1938, however, they reported success in children up to the age of 14 [38].

Robb and Steinberg, in 1938, introduced the use of ether and cyanide circulation times as a guide to the timing of successive exposures in order to obtain sequential opacification of the right and left heart [41]. Their technique was applicable to adults, and they further suggested the possibility of utilizing cineroentgenography and rapid serial roentgenography and of coordinating the exposure with the heartbeat [42]. By January 1939, they were able to report on 238 injections made in 127 patients, of whom 42 were normal, 47 had pulmonary disease, and 38 had heart disease [43]. They found that angiocardiography could differentiate between prominent pulmonary vessels and mediastinal or hilar masses, and that the technique could demonstrate characteristic changes in congenital, rheumatic, pulmonary, hypertensive, and luetic heart disease as well. As a result of their independent contributions, angiocardiography became a more versatile and reliable diagnostic tool, permitting opacification of all four cardiac chambers and the great vessels.

Sussman and his group in New York, meanwhile, were exploring the possibilities of angiocardiography in congenital and acquired heart disease, and in August 1941 they published the first of a series of excellent papers.

They illustrated the first angiocardiographic diagnosis of a case of tetralogy of Fallot in the American literature, defined the different types of dextrocardia, presented criteria for the diagnosis of patent ductus arteriosus and intracardiac shunts, and designed a practical device for multiple exposures during angiocardiography [44–47].

From 1943 until about 1947, there was a hiatus in the literature on angiocardiography in congenital heart disease, and few significant contributions appeared. Castellanos and his group continued to elaborate on some of their previously published material [48, 49], and in 1948 published a volume on congenital heart disease in which they summarized their clinical knowledge, their angiocardiographic findings, and their experience with retrograde aortography [50]. In 1947, Chavez and his co-workers described in detail a technique for intracardiac angiocardiography, injecting the opaque medium directly into the heart through a catheter [51]. Jönsson and his associates used this method of 'selective' angiocardiography extensively and obtained excellent opacification of the cardiac chambers [52, 53].

Dotter and Steinberg, meanwhile, were intensively investigating the applications of angiocardiography to pulmonary and cardiac disease in adults [54], and in 1951 published an excellent volume on angiocardiography summarizing their experience [55]. This comprehensive monograph dealt lucidly and in detail with technique, normal configurations in adults, and abnormalities detectable in cardiac, pulmonary, and mediastinal disease.

In the same year, De Groot reported his experience in a monograph describing a limited number of cases of congenital heart disease studied by angiocardiography [56], and Robb published *An Atlas of Angiocardiography* [57]. Carson and his co-workers, Colley and Sloan, Campbell and Hills, and others also made impressive contributions during this period [58–66].

The development of thoracic aortography paralleled that of angiocardiography. Using the direct-puncture technique which had been applied to animals, Nuvoli in 1936 studied the aorta in man, showing aneurysm, tortuosity, and other conditions [67]. Countercurrent or retrograde brachial aortography was described in 1939 by Castellanos and Pereiras [68], and catheter aortography by Radner in 1948 [69].

With the introduction of the percutaneous transfemoral catherization method in 1953, by Seldinger, the groundwork of the modern method of studying patent ductus arteriosus and coarctation angiographically was well established [70] (Fig. 6).

Technical advances during this period included the development of a rapid film changer by Gidlund [71] and of biplane film changers by Axen and Lind [72], the application of cineangiocardiography [73, 74], and the movement toward practical image amplification suggested by Chamberlain in 1942 [75] and subsequently developed by Coltman in 1948 [76] and Sturm and Morgan

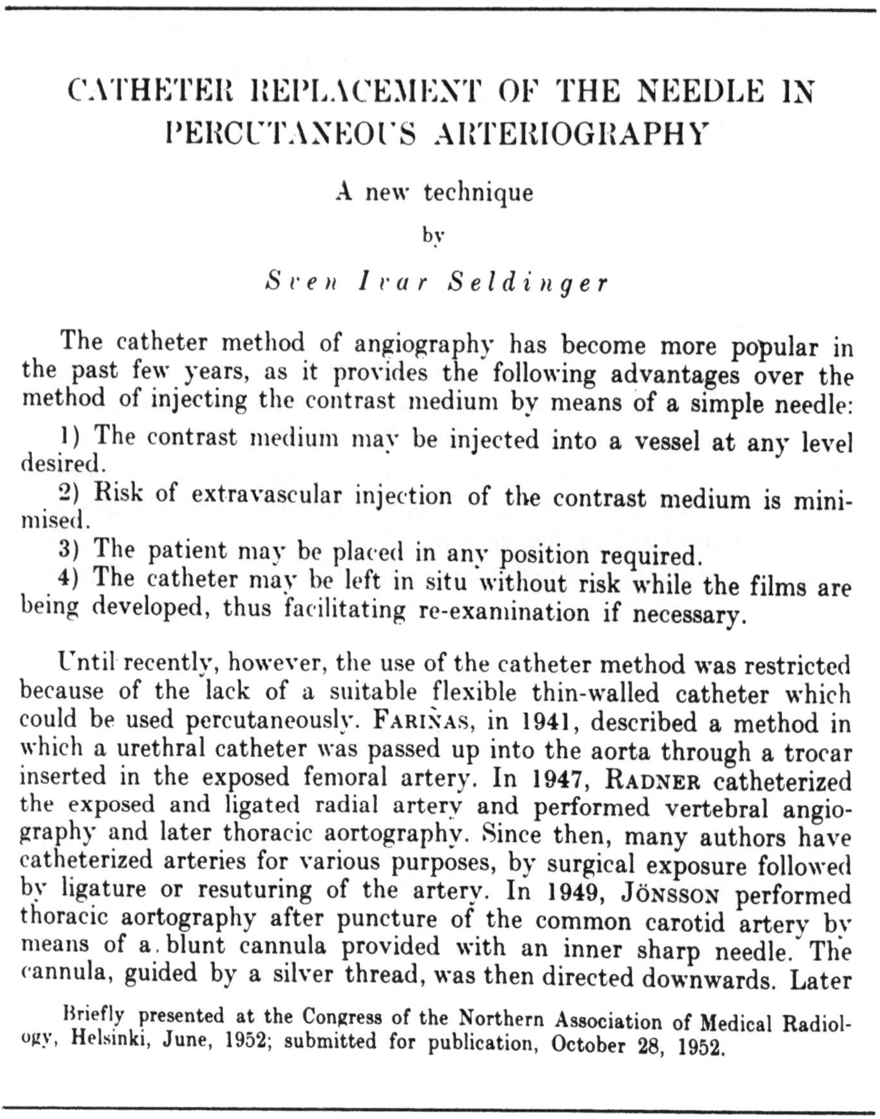

CATHETER REPLACEMENT OF THE NEEDLE IN PERCUTANEOUS ARTERIOGRAPHY

A new technique

by

Sven Ivar Seldinger

The catheter method of angiography has become more popular in the past few years, as it provides the following advantages over the method of injecting the contrast medium by means of a simple needle:

1) The contrast medium may be injected into a vessel at any level desired.

2) Risk of extravascular injection of the contrast medium is minimised.

3) The patient may be placed in any position required.

4) The catheter may be left in situ without risk while the films are being developed, thus facilitating re-examination if necessary.

Until recently, however, the use of the catheter method was restricted because of the lack of a suitable flexible thin-walled catheter which could be used percutaneously. FARIÑAS, in 1941, described a method in which a urethral catheter was passed up into the aorta through a trocar inserted in the exposed femoral artery. In 1947, RADNER catheterized the exposed and ligated radial artery and performed vertebral angiography and later thoracic aortography. Since then, many authors have catheterized arteries for various purposes, by surgical exposure followed by ligature or resuturing of the artery. In 1949, JÖNSSON performed thoracic aortography after puncture of the common carotid artery by means of a blunt cannula provided with an inner sharp needle. The cannula, guided by a silver thread, was then directed downwards. Later

Briefly presented at the Congress of the Northern Association of Medical Radiology, Helsinki, June, 1952; submitted for publication, October 28, 1952.

Fig. 6. Introduction of the percutaneous transfemoral catheterization method in 1953 by Seldinger.

in 1949 [77]. Chapman and his co-workers described the use of biplane cine-fluorography to evaluate ventricular volume in 1958 [78] and, in the same year, Abrams introduced biplane image amplified cineangiocardiography [79], which has since become the most widely applied method of studying children with congenital heart disease.

The final major episode was the development of coronary arteriography in

26

man, first described by Gunnar Jönsson in 19418 [80], amplified by Dotter and Frische with aortic occlusion in 1958 [81], and finally applied to man as a selective technique in 1959 by F. Mason Sones [82] (Fig. 7). In 1961, Ricketts and Abrams first performed percutaneous transfemoral selective coronary

A MONTHLY SCIENTIFIC PUBLICATION OF THE AMERICAN HEART ASSOCIATION, INC.

MODERN CONCEPTS OF CARDIOVASCULAR DISEASE

Copyright© 1962 by the AMERICAN HEART ASSOCIATION, INC., 44 EAST 23rd STREET, NEW YORK 10, N.Y.
Editor: E. COWLES ANDRUS, M.D.   Associate Editor: RICHARD S. ROSS, M.D.
Editorial Office: JOHNS HOPKINS HOSPITAL, BALTIMORE 5, MARYLAND

Vol. XXXI   JULY 1962   No. 7

Cine Coronary Arteriography *

■ F. Mason Sones, Jr., M.D.
Earl K. Shirey, M.D.

*Department of Pediatric Cardiology
and Cardiac Laboratory
Cleveland Clinic
Cleveland, Ohio*

During the past four years, the technique of cine coronary arteriography has been developed in an effort to provide a more objective and precise standard of diagnosis for human coronary artery disease. Heretofore, the diagnosis of coronary atherosclerosis has been primarily dependent on the physician's interpretation of the efforts of distressed patients to describe chest pain, and upon recognition of transient or chronic electrocardiographic changes which usually indicate the presence of myocardial ischemia or necrosis. Although conscientious, knowledgeable, history-taking and electrocardiographic study require no apologist for their contributions to understanding, their limitations have been responsible, even in the hands of experts, for the production of iatrogenic disability on the one hand, and unjustified reassurance on the other, in a significant number of patients. A safe and dependable method for demonstrating the physical characteristics of the human coronary artery tree, which could be applied in any phase of the natural history of coronary artery disease, was needed to supplement available diagnostic methods.

* From the Department of Pediatric Cardiology and Cardiac Laboratory, Cleveland Clinic, Cleveland, Ohio.

Direct coronary artery catheterization has been used for deliberate selective opacification of individual coronary arteries in more than 1,020 patients. The results obtained in a characteristic group of patients are demonstrated in a motion picture entitled: "Cine Coronary Arteriography," prepared for distribution by the Committee on Professional Education of the American Heart Association in September 1962. Preliminary studies performed in our laboratory from 1956 through the first six months of 1958 on dogs and humans without clinical evidence of coronary artery disease have demonstrated that dependable opacification of the normal coronary artery tree could not be achieved by conventional aortographic techniques. Doses of contrast media, ranging from 40 to 60 cc., were injected into the aortic root under pressures of 10 Kg./cm.^{1} with a Gidlund pressure syringe, and provided adequate visualization of major branches of the right and left coronary arteries in fewer than 70 per cent of the patients studied.[1]

The use of acetylcholine to produce asystole and facilitate improved coronary perfusion with smaller doses of contrast media was explored by Lehman and associates.[1] This seemed undesirable because of the variable response of different patients to similar doses of the drug, and because we feared the consequences of its use in patients with unknown degrees of myocardial ischemia.

Dotter and associates[1] proposed the introduction of a balloon catheter into the ascending aorta to produce temporary aortic occlusion, while injecting a small dose of contrast sub-

---

Fig. 7. Selective coronary arteriography applied to man in 1959 by F. Mason Sones.

27

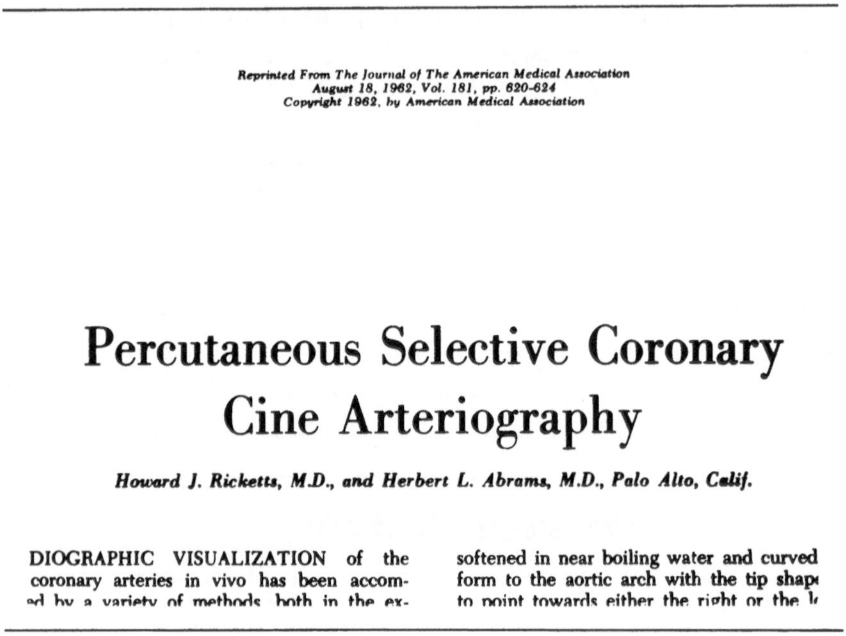

Reprinted From The Journal of The American Medical Association
August 18, 1962, Vol. 181, pp. 820-624
Copyright 1962, by American Medical Association

Percutaneous Selective Coronary Cine Arteriography

Howard J. Ricketts, M.D., and Herbert L. Abrams, M.D., Palo Alto, Calif.

DIOGRAPHIC VISUALIZATION of the coronary arteries in vivo has been accom-
~d by a variety of methods, both in the ex-

softened in near boiling water and curved
form to the aortic arch with the tip shap~
to point towards either the right or the l~

Fig. 8. Ricketts and Abrams first perform percutaneous transfemoral selective coronary arteriography with preformed catheters (1961).

arteriography with preformed catheters [83] (Fig. 8), and five years later Judkins modified transfemoral preformed catheters with thermoplastic material to
provide what has today become the most widely applied method of coronary
arteriography throughout the world [84].

No sophisticated surgery has ever been able to develop in the history of
modern medicine without a preceding sophisticated radiology to provide a
road map. This is as true of surgery of the brain, lungs, gastrointestinal tract,
kidneys, and bone as it is of the cardiovascular system. By the time open
heart surgery became feasible in the mid 1950s, angiocardiography had grad-
uated from the status of an experimental investigative procedure with little
clinical applicability to a highly refined diagnostic method. It was thus able
immediately to be put to use to provide for the surgeon the kind of morpho-
logic information which was essential not only to successful surgery at the
time, but to the development of new methods of handling more and more
complicated lesions.

Improvements in angiocardiography have been designed to decrease the
dangers and improve the quality of the studies. As a consequence, new media
have been synthesized, and meticulous preangiographic and postangiographic
care have become a central and important focus. These complex and
immensely revealing diagnostic procedures can be performed in 1979 with a

28

minimum of hazard to the patient and with a maximum of critical information on which to base the clinical management of the patient. We all owe a great debt of gratitude to Drs. Castellanos and Steinberg for their pioneering contributions to diagnostic medicine.

REFERENCES

1. Roentgen WC (1895) On a new kind of rays. Erste Mitt Sitzber Phys Med Ges (Wurzburg) 137
2. Glasser O (1934) Wilhelm Conrad Roentgen and the early history of the X-rays. Springfield IL: Thomas
3. Becher W (1896) Zur Anwendung des roentgenischen Verfahrens in der Medizin. Dtsch Med Wochenschr 22:202
4. Cannon WB (1898) The movements of the stomach studied by means of the roentgen ray. Am J Physiol 1:359
5. Haschek E, Lindenthal OT (1896) A contribution to the practical use of the photography according to Röntgen. Wien Klin Wochenschr 9:63
6. Morton WG, Hammer EW (1896) The X-ray, or, photography of the invisible and its value in surgery. New York: American Technical
7. Voelcker F, Lichtenberg A (1906) Pyelographie (Röntgenographie des Nierenbeckens nach Kollargolfüllung). Munch Med Wochenschr 53:105
8. Orrin HC (1920) The X-ray atlas of the systemic arteries of the body. London: Baillière, Tindall, and Cox
9. Franck O, Alwens W (1910) Kreislaufstudien am Röntgenschirm. Munch Med Wochenschr 51:950
10. Sicard JA, Forestier G (1923) Injections intravasculaires d'huile iodée sous controle radiologique. CR Soc Biol (Paris) 88:1200
11. Berberich J, Hirsch S (1923) Die Röntgenographische Darstellung der Arterien und Venen am Lebenden. Munch Klin Wochenschr 18:2226
12. Brooks B (1924) Intraarterial injection of sodium iodide. JAMA 82:1016
13. Carnett JB, Greenbaum SS (1927) Blood vessel visualization. JAMA 89:2039
14. Saito M, Kamikawa K, Yanagizawa K (1930) Blood vessel visualization in vivo. Am J Surg 10:225
15. Charbonnel and Massé (1929) Artériographie des membres avec l'iodure de sodium, spécialment dans les artérites. Bull Mem Soc Natl Chir 55:735
16. Moniz E, Diaz A, Lima A (1928) La radioartériographie et la topographie cranioencephalique. J Radiol Electr 12:72
17. Forssmann W (1931) Über Kontrastdarstellung der Höhlen des levenden rechten Herzens und der Lungenschlagader. Munch Med Wochenschr 78:489
18. dos Santos R, Lamas AC, Pereira-Caldas J (1929) Arteriografia da aorta e dos vasos abdominais. Med Contemp 47:93
19. Moniz E, de Carvalho L, Lima A (1931) Angiopneumographie. Presse Med 53:996
20. Binz A (1937) Geschichte des Uroselectans. Z Urol 31:73
21. Binz A, Rath C (1928) Über biochemische Eigenschaften von Derivaten des Pyridins und Chinolins. Biochem Z 203:218
22. Swick N (1929) Darstellung der Niere und Harnwege in Röntgenbild durch intravenöse Einbringung eines neuen Kontraststoffes, des Uroselectans. Klin Wochenschr 8:2087
23. Pearse HE, Warren SL (1931) The röntgenographic visualization of the arteries of the extremities in peripheral vascular disease. Ann Surg 94:1094

24. Schüller J (1931) Zweijährige Erfahrung mit der Arteriographie. Arch Orthop Unfallchir 30:233

25. Frey S, Zwerg HG (1931) Die röntgenologische Darstellung der Gefässe am lebenden Eiere und Menschen. (Vasographie.) Dtsch Z Chir 232:173

26. Wohlleben T (1932) Venographie. Klin Wochenschr 112:1786

27. Barber THT, Orley A (1932) Some x-ray observations in varicose disease of the leg. Lancet 2:175

28. Edwards EA (1933) The status of vasography. N Engl J Med 209:1337

29. Rousthöi P (1933) Über Angiokardiographie. Acta Radiol (Stockholm) 14:119

30. Conte E, Costa A (1933) Angiopneumography. Radiology 21:461

31. Ravina A (1934) L'exploration radiologique des vaisseaux pulmonaires par l'injection de substances de contraste. Prog Med (Paris) 3:1701

32. Reboul H, Racine M (1933) La ventriculographie cardiaque expérimentale. Presse Med 41:763

33. Ameuille P, Ronneaux G, Hinault V, Desgrez, Lemoine JM (1936) Remarques sur quelques cas d'artériographie pulmonaire chez l'homme vivant. Bull Mem Soc Med Hop Paris 52:729

34. Castellanos A, Pereiras R, Garcia A (1937) La angiocardiografia radio-opaca. Arch Soc Estud Clin (Habana) 31:523

35. Cardelle G, Sanchez-Santiago B, Castellanos A, Pereiras R (1938) Tronco arterial común persistente; su diagnóstico intra-vitam por la angiocardiografia. Bol Soc Cubana Pediatr 10:247

36. Castellanos A (1938) Sobre el diagnóstico angio-cardiográfico de la communicación inter-ventricular. Arch Latino Am Cardiol Hematol 8:1

37. Castellanos A, Pereiras R, Garcia A (1938) Angio-cardiographies in newborn. Bol Soc Cubana Pediatr 10:225

38. Castellanos A, Pereiras R, Garcia A, Vasquez-Paussa A (1938) On the factors intervening in the obtention of perfect angiocardiograms. Bol Soc Cubana Pediatr 10:217

39. Castellanos A, Pereiras R, Lopez AY (1938) La angio-cardiografía. Rev Cien Med 1:1

40. Castellanos A, Pereiras R, Vasquez-Paussa A (1938) On a special automatic device for angio-cardiography. Bol Soc Cubana Pediatr 10:209

41. Robb GP, Steinberg I (1938) A practical method of visualization of chambers of the heart, the pulmonary circulation, and the great blood vessels in man. J Clin Invest 17:507

42. Robb GP, Steinberg I (1939) Visualization of the chambers of the heart, the pulmonary circulation, and the great blood vessels in man. Am J Roentgenol 41:1

43. Robb GP, Steinberg I (1939) Visualization of the chambers of the heart, the pulmonary circulation, and the great blood vessels in heart disease. Preliminary observations. Am J Roentgenol 42:14

44. Steinberg MF, Grishman A, Sussman ML (1942) Angiocardiography in congenital heart disease. I. Dextrocardia. Am J Roentgenol 48:141

45. Steinberg MF, Grishman A, Sussman ML (1943) Angiocardiography in congenital heart disease. II. Intracardiac shunts. Am J Roentgenol 49:766

46. Steinberg MF, Grishman, Sussman ML (1943) Angiocardiography in congenital heart disease. III. Patent ductus arteriosus. Am J Roentgenol 50:306

47. Sussman ML, Steinberg MF, Grishman A (1941) Multiple exposure technique in contrast visualization of the cardiac chambers and great vessels. Am J Roentgenol 46:745

48. Castellanos A, Lopez AG, Pereiras R (1945) Sobre la radio-opacificación de las cavidades izquierdas del corazón, de la aorta y sus ramas (levo-angiocardiograma); su importancia practica. Rev Cubana Cardiol 6:87

49. Castellanos A, Pereiras R, Lopez AG (1945) Arco Aórtico a la derecha en el niño. Estudio general. Valor de la angiocardiografía. Arch Inst Cardiol Mex 15:301

50. Castellanos A, Cabrera L (1948) Cardiopatias Congenitas de la Infancia. Havana: Publicaciónes Cientifilas
51. Chavez I, Dorbecker N, Celis A (1947) Direct intracardiac angiocardiography: its diagnostic value. Am Heart J 33:560
52. Jönsson G (1951) Selective visualization in angiocardiography. J Fac Radiol 3:125
53. Jönsson G, Broden B, Karnell J (1949) Selective angiocardiography. Acta Radiol 32:486
54. Dotter CT, Steinberg I (1950) Advances in angiocardiography. Med Clin North Am 34:745
55. Dotter CT, Steinberg I (1951) Angiocardiography. New York: Paul Hoeber
56. De Groot JWC (1951) Angiocardiography as a diagnostic aid in congenital heart disease. Amsterdam: Keesing
57. Robb GP (1951) An atlas of angiocardiography. American Registry of Pathology
58. Axén O, Lind J (1950) Electrocardiographic recording in angiocardiography with synchronous serial photography at right-angled planes. Cardiologia 16:61
59. Campbell M, Hills TH (1950) Angiocardiography in cyanotic congenital heart disease. Br Heart J 12:65
60. Carson MJ, Burford TH, Scott WG, Goodfriend J (1948) Diagnosis of pulmonary stenosis by angiocardiography. J Pediatr 33:525
61. Cooley RN, Bahnson HT, Hanlon CR (1949) Angiocardiography in congenital heart disease of cyanotic type with pulmonic stenosis or atresia: observations on the tetralogy of Fallot and 'pseudo-truncus arteriosus'. Radiology 52:329
62. Cooley RN, Sloan RD (1952) Angiocardiography and congenital heart disease of cyanotic type: observations on complete transposition of the great vessels. Radiology 58:481
63. Cooley RN, Sloan RD, Hanlon CR, Bahnson HT (1950) Angiocardiography in congenital heart disease of cyanotic type: observations on tricuspid atresia or atresia with hypoplasia of right ventricle. Radiology 54:848
64. Gasul BM, Weiss H, Fell EH, Dillon RF, Fisher DL, Marienfeld CJ (1953) Angiocardiography in congenital heart disease correlated with clinical and autopsy findings. AMA Am J Dis Child 85:404
65. Kreutzer RO, Caprile JA, Wessels FM (1950) Angiocardiography in heart disease in children. Br Heart J 12:293
66. Lind J, Wegellus C (1950) New trends in angiocardiography. Med Illustr 4:1
67. Nuvoli I (1936) Arteriografia dell'aorta toracica mediante punctura dell'aorta ascendente o del ventriculos. Policlinico (Prat) 43:227
68. Radner S (1948) Thoracic aortography by catheterization from the radial artery. Acta Radiol (Stockholm) 29:178
69. Castellanos A, Pereiras R (1939) Counter-current aortography. Rev Cuba Cariol 2:187
70. Seldinger SI (1953) Catheter replacement of needle in percutaneous arteriography: new technique. Acta Radiol 39:368–376
71. Gidlund AS (1949) New apparatus for direct cineroentgenography. Acta Radiol 32:81–88
72. Axen O, Lind J (1950) Electrocardiographic recording in angiocardiography with synchronous serial photography at right angled planes. Cardiologia 16:60–66
73. Janker R, Hallerbach H (1951) Die angiocardiokinematographie als Mittel zur Bestimmung der Lungenkreislaufzeit. Fortschr Roentgenstr 75:290
74. Ramsey GHS, Watson JS Jr, Steinhausen TB, Thompson JJ, Dreisinger F, Weinberg S (1949) Cinefluorography: a progress report on technical problems, dosage factors, and clinical impressions. Radiology 52:684
75. Chamberlain WE (1942) Fluoroscopes and fluoroscopy; Carman lecture. Radiology 38:383–413
76. Coltman JW (1948) Fluoroscopic image brightening by electronic means. Radiology 51:359–366

77. Sturm RE, Morgan RH (1949) Screen intensification systems and their limitations. Am J Roentgenol 62:617–634
78. Chapman CB, Baker O, Reynolds J, et al. (1958) Use of biplane cinefluorography for measurement of ventricular volume. Circulation 18:1105–1117
79. Abrams HL (1958, 1959) An approach to biplane cineangiocardiography. Radiology 72:735–740, 741–750; 73:531–538
80. Jönsson G (1948) Visualization of the coronary arteries: preliminary report. Acta Radiol 29:536–540
81. Dotter CT, Frische LH (1958) Visualization of the coronary circulation by occlusion aortography: a practical method. Radiology 71:502–524
82. Sones FM Jr, Shirey EK (1962) Cine coronary arteriography. Mod Conc Cardiovasc Dis 31:735–738
83. Ricketts HJ, Abrams HL (1962) Percutaneous selective coronary cinearteriography. JAMA 181:620–624
84. Judkins MP (1967) Selective coronary arteriography, a percutaneous transfemoral technique. Radiology 89:815–824

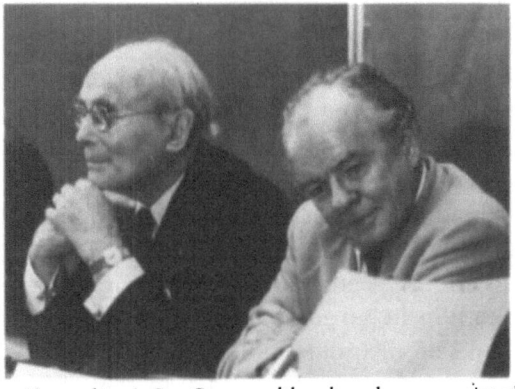

A. J. DUNNING

André Frédéric Cournand (left), born in Paris in 1895, received his medical degree there. From 1930, he worked in Bellevue Hospital, New York, together with Dickinson W. Richards on pulmonary pathophysiology. This involved the pulmonary circulation, which they studied by using and perfecting the technique of heart catheterization, first used for this purpose by Marey and Chauveau in the horse and dog, and by Werner Forssmann in man (with himself as subject). Dr. Cournand has long been associated with the Columbia University, College of Physicians and Surgeons, and is still with the College as a special lecturer.

F. Mason Sones (right) was director of the cardiac laboratory (from 1950 till 1966) and later of the department of cardiovascular diseases (from 1966 till 1975) at the Cleveland Clinic Foundation, which he is still serving as senior physician. His chief interest lies in the combination of cardiac catheterization with cineangiography to arrive at the diagnosis of cardiovascular disease. Since 1959, he has made a major contribution by developing selective coronary arteriography and demonstrating its feasibility and value.

Interview with André Cournand at Leiden, November 1979

D: I would like to take you back, Dr. Cournand, to the beginning of your investigations. When I was a young cardiologist in training, my first tool in hand was a Cournand catheter and your name is still a household word. However, you did not start with a tool but with a concept. You decided, together with that remarkable Dr. Dickinson Richards, to start an investigation of cardiorespiratory function.

C: More exactly, respiratory function in disease as well as in normal men. It was the application of physiological methods, already known or under development, to the study of pulmonary function in its various aspects. These can be divided very grossly now, but at that time we knew exactly how much we had to study in ventilation, its distribution through the lung, diffusion and, after that, the transfer through the lung of blood from the right side of the heart to the left ventricle.

D: At that time it probably was a daring concept. You started with the physiologist Henderson, did your work in two laboratories in two different hospitals, and from the onset set your target high.

C: Yes, but at the time a superb amount of work had been done by Swedish, Danish, British, and American investigators in the physiology of respiration, by men like Liljestrand, Haldane, Henderson, and Van Slyke in the United States. But we added something important, which could only be revealed in desease: the relationship between alveolar ventilation and perfusion. The lead was given to us very early in our study on the basis of the application of the Fick principle, when we were trying to equilibrate the blood content of carbon dioxide to the alveolar, that is the pulmonary, content of carbon dioxide. That involved equilibrium and the certainty of reaching it. That was possible with the rebreathing method in normal subjects when you reached equilibrium in seven seconds. In disease you could not reach that because of uneven distribution. That actually led us from the study of cardiac output and pulmonary blood flow to something quite different: the unequal distribution of blood flow in disease. That brought us to a new method, the use of nitrogen and its washout by pure oxygen, the curve of this washout indicating how the gas was distributed during successive ventilations.

D: What you were looking for was the mixed venous blood and its oxygen content?

C: We were to apply the Fick principle. At the same time we measured the carbon dioxide output and carbon dioxide content of the arterial blood. But the mixed venous blood equilibration was based on gas tension, thus we had to reach equilibrium, then referred the pressure to a curve giving us the carbon dioxide concentration, and then we had to correct for the pure oxygen that we were using at that time for the equilibration. Very complicated and time-consuming. It took us one whole day to do one measurement of cardiac output.

D: Before you started with volunteers and patients in shock, you did some work on animals like dogs and chimpanzees?

C: In 1932, when we established our program with Dickinson Richards, he asked: 'Would not it be nice to get mixed venous blood directly?' Then he got the article of Forssmann, published in 1929, and he said: 'The catheter is the answer,' but we were not ready to use it. It was only in 1936 that we used it, after we had realized that we could not reach equilibrium in pulmonary disease. So I went to Paris and, as you probably know, I did nearly all my training there, in hospital, to finish what is equivalent to a residency, as *interne des hôpitaux*. I completed training in medicine in all its forms but with a particular interest in pulmonary disease. Although my thesis was on acute disseminated sclerosis, a neurological subject, my real interest was lung disease.

I went to the united States to spend one year in a clinic of pulmonary disease and in the Trudeau sanatorium, which was one of the best in the world at that time. Then, in 1966, I went to see an old teacher of mine,

Ameuille, who published as the first French investigator on pulmonary angiography.

They had a very rough time at the Société Médical des Hôpitaux de Paris, and all the best-known cardiologists advised them to stop that kind of study, as they told McMichael later.

There was a Paris physician by the name of André Ravinat, who had written about cardiac catheterization, examined a report on 100 cases of angiography, and found out that, being very careful, there was no trouble at all and they had fine pictures. I went back to New York. I had to do my work on gas analysis in blood and air in the bacteriology lab, because we had a lack of space. My Haldane and the Van Slyke apparatus stood there. Then, at the same time, Steinberg and Robb were working in that same laboratory on preparing concentrated iodine solutions as a contrast medium. We had a silk catheter (obtained in Paris) which could be passed through a needle, and there were Steinberg and Robb devising a method of contrast angiography which could eliminate the necessity of an angiography catheter.

D: When you had that catheter, you used it to full advantage. Once having the tool, you explored several categories of disease.

C: I would emphasize that we had a problem to solve, like Chauveau and Marey and, before them, Claude Bernard; they used a new technique to solve it. For Chauveau, it was finding the site of heat production in tissue; for Marey, it was the timing of the apex beat. What we wanted was to study pulmonary circulation in diseases of the lung and we needed therefore a good measurement of flow. In 1936, we started with a young resident, Robert C. Darling, on our work in dogs, which took us four years. Then we studied a chimpanzee which was lent to us by someone who was trying to find a vaccine against influenza.

D: A costly present then?

C: Yes it was, and that chimpanzee was the first case in which we studied pulmonary edema. During the same time, George Wright, who was a pulmonary physiologist and had been working in Cleveland under Wiggers, studied in the autopsy room the relation between the right atrium and a reference point on the thorax as a landmark. This point, five centimeters under the angle of Louis, served as reference point for measurement of pressure in the heart. The question was what the true zero point had to be. Of course the heart lies in the thorax and we don't know what the intrathoracic pressure is which should be subtracted.

Then, in 1940, we were ready for our study in man. We could measure intracardiac pressures by saline manometers and determine cardiac output, based on the Fick principle, by sampling blood and air in a safe procedure, both in normal men and later in patients in shock and congestive heart failure. We published our first report in 1941 and the rest of the study is known.

D: What amazes me, Dr. Cournand, is the following. You are now 83 years old, and retired from active practice some 20 years ago. But 10 years ago you edited a book called *Shaping the Future*. You look backward and forward.

C: I did not write it; I edited it with my friend, Dr. Maurice Levy. It happened that in 1957 in Paris I met a philosopher, Gaston Berger, then working in the Ministry of Higher Education in France. He had written an extremely important article in the New French Encyclopedia on what he described as prospective thinking. It dealt with operational time, an idea derived from Maurice Blondel. The future is unknown but it is not the continuation of the past. Future is created by man and the present should be studied by anticipating the future. That is a reversal of the usual order of past, present, and future. By imaging the future we can study the present, which may be pregnant of developments to come. To use your imagination of what is favorable to man in the future, you can base your decisions for today.

This notion is dynamic and leads to the conclusion that the future image will be modified as soon as you change the present. There is a continuous adaptation, if you like, to our idea of the future. Is that notion of perspective developed in Holland? In France it has a great influence not only in philosophy but in all thinking on the future, in government planning, industry, and science.

D: Dr. Cournand, you are not only a medical man but you have a deep and long-standing interest in philosophy, in the ethics of science, and your collaborator, Dr. Dickinson Richards, was an excellent Greek scholar.

C: Yes, we continued working together after 1965, after our retirement. We set up a program for medical schools, which dealt with the history of medicine and its relation to society. Dickinson Richards and Fishman were asked by the NIH to prepare a book on the history of the study of the circulation, about men and ideas. Our program was pretty unique, because we had senior scientists who came to medical school and lectured on their work some twenty/thirty years ago. The students actually met the people who wrote part of the history of medicine. René Dubos gave several lectures and published those in a book. Dickinson Richards directed several seminars and I talked on medicine and society. We had small groups of nurses and young assistants, hospital administrators, young activists, discussing medical education. These ideas discussed by volunteers outside the curriculum were then formally introduced in teaching programs on ethics, history, and the humanities in the medical school. Students are often not interested in things not directly related to patient care, but the humanities shape the man.

D: Dr. Cournand, let me pose my last question. Is there any age at which an active scientist should retire?

C: I have not finished yet and, as you know, I have been busy by working on the code of the scientist for five or six years. I try to develop the notion that the ethical code of the scientist could give an example of what human behavior should be in a changing society. Perspective, ethics, the relation of medicine to society are things which have my interest. The essential thing about the code of the scientist is that it forms the code of the honest man. He is intellectually honest, he judges on the basis of objectivity, as fast as one can judge by objective standards, he is tolerant of other people's ideas, he recognizes errors, he is on his guard toward authoritarianism and certitudes, and is disinterested. I believe this is what makes science universal and could provide a code of ethics for all men. This is not to disparage the fact that we are also moved by emotions, but we should disregard them when making decisions.

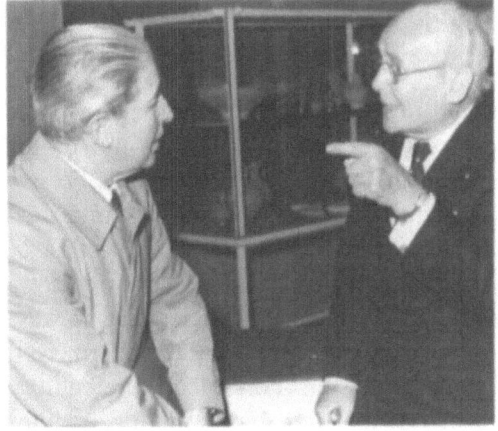

FRANZ LOOGEN

F. Loogen (left) and A. F. Cournand (right) discussing the heart of the matter in the National Museum of Antiquities, Leiden. Franz Loogen is head of the cardiological department and professor of medicine at the University Hospital of Düsseldorf. He has done a great deal of work on the preoperative and postoperative evaluation of patients with valvular and congenital heart lesions.

In memory of Werner Forssmann

Werner Forssmann was born in Berlin on August 28th, 1904. When he finished his medical studies in 1928, he wanted to specialize in internal medicine, but did not succeed in getting an appropriate position. Therefore, he started training as surgeon and urologist at the small Auguste Victoria Hospital in Eberswalde near Berlin. The head of the Hospital was Dr. Schneider, an old family friend.

Meanwhile, Forssmann continued to be interested in internal medicine. However, while he focused on cardiac diseases, he became disappointed with the insufficient diagnostic and therapeutic possibilities. Thinking of new diagnostic means, he was attracted by the idea to introduce a catheter into the heart. His thinking was decisively influenced by the experimental studies by Claude Bernard and by Chauveau and Marey in the years between 1854 and 1863. In his memoirs, Forssmann says: 'Already at the beginning of my medical studies I was fascinated by the works of Claude Bernard, Chauveau and Marey. I hoped that it should be possible to transfer this procedure to man.'

He mentioned his ideas to his chief and asked for permission to do the experiment on himself. But Dr. Schneider replied in horror, 'For heaven's sake, don't be a fool. Drop this suicidal idea. What could I tell your mother if one day we should find you dead?'

In spite of this, the very obstinate Forssmann pursued his ideas. With the aid of a colleague, Dr. Romeis, a thick needle was introduced into an arm vein. Through this, a well-oiled ureteral catheter was passed up to a distance of 35 cm. At this moment, Dr. Romeis refused to go further, fearing that the experiment might end fatally.

Forssmann did not give up; he decided to repeat the procedure alone. One week after the failed attempt, he ordered the 'senior operating nurse' to prepare instruments for a patient to have an ureteral catheterization. Forssmann told the nurse that he did not want further assistance, so the nurse left the room. Then, suspicious, she returned and found Forssmann injecting a local anesthetic into his own left antecubital fossa. It is well known how Forssman succeeded in persuading the nurse. He explained to her that he was merely going to pass a catheter into a vein and that this would be harmless. The nurse then insisted on having it done on herself. Forssmann, pretending to go along with her, strapped her arm down while she was lying on the operating table. But with his back toward the nurse, he opened his own left cephalic vein and introduced the ureteral catheter up to 30 cm. With the catheter in his arm and with the assistance of the nurse, who had wiggled herself free in the meantime, Forssmann walked through a long corridor, then down two flights of stairs to the X-ray department. Here he stepped behind a fluoroscopic screen. With the nurse holding a mirror in front of the screen, he was able to follow the progress of the catheter from the left subclavian region into the right heart. Forssmann insisted on having a photographic record, as he was afraid that no one would believe him. This picture appeared in his original publication in 1929 in the *Klinische Wochenschrift*, entitled: 'Die Sondierung des rechten Herzens.'

After his publication, Forssmann did not receive the expected appreciation from the medical public. He even had to leave his job at the famous Charité in Berlin, which he was given shortly before the publication of his paper. In spite of these drawbacks, he continued his studies after having returned to Eberswalde. Up to 1930, he had done nine catheterizations on himself and, in a few of them, he also used contrast medium for opacification of the right ventricle and pulmonary artery. When he presented the results of his studies at the annual meeting of the German surgical society in München in April 1931, he received an icy response. There was no applause and no discussion.

Forssmann did not continue his research, but limited his activities to surgery and urology. His name and his work were forgotten until, in 1941, Cournand and Ranges published their paper on 'Catheterisation of the right auricle in man' (*Proc. Soc. Exp. Med.* 46 [1941]: 462). In this article, the authors made reference to the first attempts of Forssmann in the late 1920s. In view of his former disappointing experiences with his German colleagues, Forssmann was deeply impressed by this honorable and fair attitude. In 1956, Forssmann was awarded the Nobel Prize together with Cournand and Richards. During the last decade of his active life, Forssmann was the chief surgeon of a large hospital in Düsseldorf.

The last time I met him was during the first days of May 1979, when we

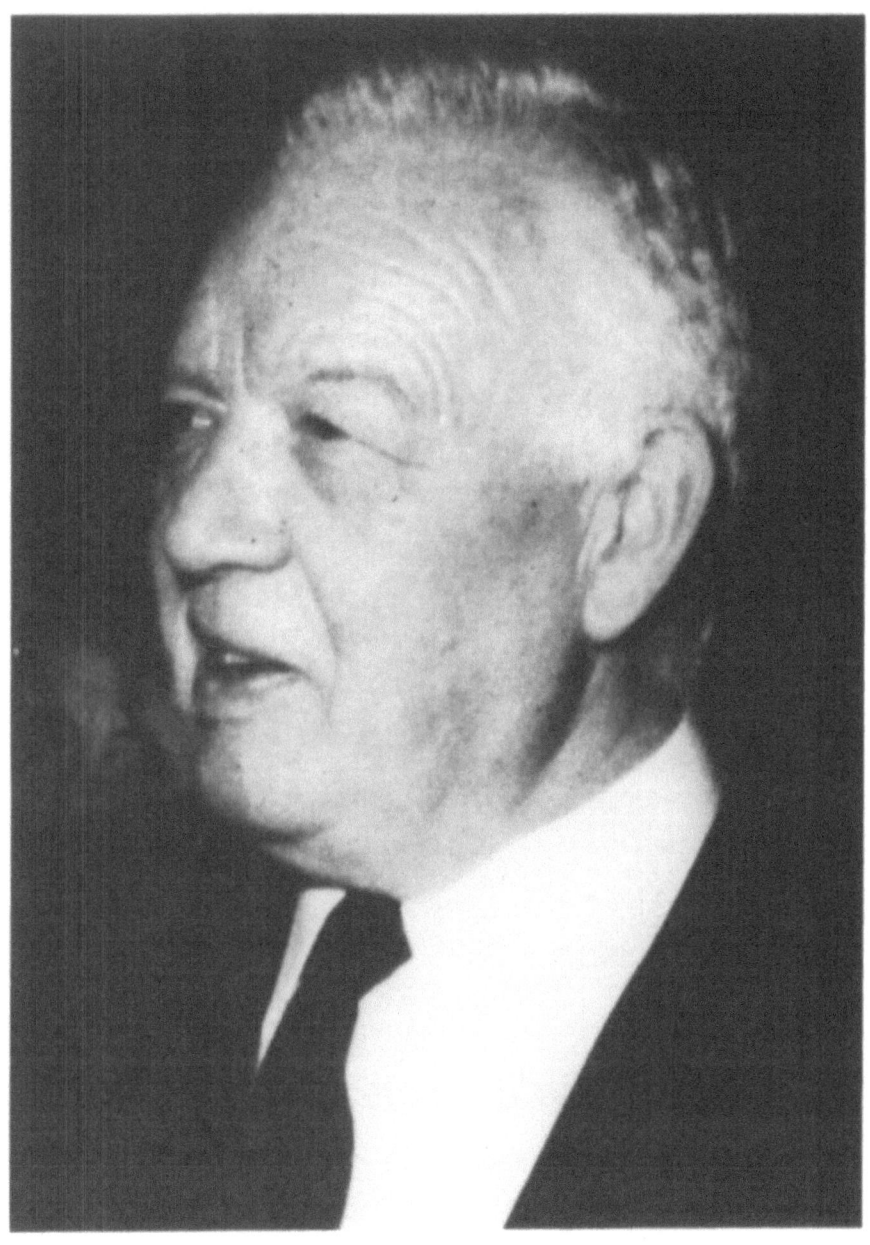

Dr. Werner Forssmann

celebrated the 30th anniversary of the first heart operation after the war in Düsseldorf. The picture above was taken on that occasion. Four weeks later (1 June 1979), Forssmann died from myocardial infarction at the age of almost 75 years.

REFERENCES

Bernard C (1855–56) Leçons de physiologie expérimentale appliquée à la médicine (Paris)
Chauveau JBA, Marey EJ (1862) De la force déployée par la contraction des différentes cavités du cœur. CR Soc Biol (Paris) 4, 3 [Ser]:131
Forssmann W (1929) Die Sondierung des rechten Herzens. Klin Wochenschr 8:2085–87
Forssmann W (1931) Über Kontrastdarstellung der Höhlen des lebenden rechten Herzens und der Lungenschlagader. Munch Med Wochenschr 1:489–492

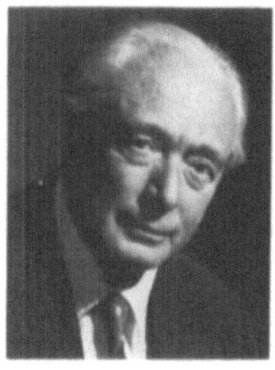

RICHARD J. BING

Richard J. Bing was born 1909, and after finishing his medical studies in Europe, held teaching appointments at Johns Hopkins and was professor of medicine at various American universities. He presently is attached to the University of Southern California School of Medicine. His major contribution to cardiology is the study of cardiac metabolism, carried out in the experimental animal and in the catheterization laboratory. Most of this work was done in the 1950s at the University of Alabama.

Personal memories of cardiac catheterization and metabolism of the heart

When I was in the army, I received in the summer of 1945 a telephone call from Alfred Blalock, Chairman of the Department of Surgery at the Johns Hopkins Hospital, asking me whether I would be willing to set up a physiological laboratory for the study of congenital heart disease. It was the time when Blalock and Helen Taussig had already operated on quite a number of children with congenital heart disease. The question was purely rhetorical because the answer was obviously 'yes.' As soon as I got out of the army, I watched André Cournand for a couple of weeks to see how the famous team in New York was doing, and then went to the 'provinces' in Baltimore to set up a physiological laboratory. I should mention here that I was particularly interested in the physiology of congenital heart disease and, to a lesser degree, in the diagnosis, but as it turned out the two went hand in hand. There were a couple of methods which I had in mind, foremost of course being catheterization of the right heart, which had been pioneered by Forssmann and by Cournand and Richards, but I was primarily very interested in how these children with congenital heart disease adapted themselves to the low oxygen tension in the blood. I also felt that what we now call 'noninvasive methods' had a place in the diagnosis of congenital heart disease. So we adopted André Cournand's exercise test which related the oxygen consumed by the patient to the liters of ventilation. We were happy to find that in most children or adults with the cyanotic type of congenital heart disease, the ratio oxygen consumption/ventilation fell during exercise. We began right heart catheterization toward the end of 1945 and I can even now remember the names of the patients who were sent to us by Blalock and Taussig.

43

An episode which occurred at that time was when a couple of distinguished visitors showed up – amongst them, Sir Henry Dale – who wanted to watch the technique. Of course the catheter room was completely dark, there was no image amplification and I pushed the catheter into the heart and then turned on the fluoroscope, and to my surprise the catheter tip showed up in the lung field. This was a rather unexpected occurrence, but it was even more frightening when Sir Henry, who was standing behind me, with a very loud voice asked me whether I had made the hole myself! Obviously he thought I had punctured the heart. The difficulties at that time, in catheterization, were certainly undreamed of today with all the electronic gadgetry available. We used a Hamilton manometer which began to leak at the most crucial moments. We learned to appreciate the importance of increased pulmonary artery pressure which so often accompanies certain types of congenital heart disease. But to me, of the greatest interest was the adaptation of these children with congenital heart disease to the low oxygen tension in blood. I then appreciated very much the work of Sir Joseph Barcroft and his beautiful work on 'Lessons from High Altitudes', because the similarity of congenital heart disease to high altitude was quite obvious, primarily because the adaptation to anoxia in congenital heart disease also lay in the shape of the O_2 dissociation curve.

A year later, I pushed the catheter into what I thought was the right ventricle (that must have been the end of 1946) but when I drew the blood from the catheter it was black. This was a surprise because when we pulled the catheter back a little bit, it was of the color which one expects to find in the right ventricle. Besides, the pressure from that catheter position was low like that in the atrium while that in the right ventricle showed the typical right ventricular tracing. We soon realized, working on cadavers, that we had entered either the great cardiac vein or the coronary sinus. This opened up a whole new field for me – that of cardiac metabolism. It was a new interest and, although I continued with congenital heart disease, I forsook the old love for the new one and devoted much time to the study of cardiac metabolism. Fortunately, at that time Kety and Schmidt had developed the nitrous oxide method for the measurement of cerebral blood flow through the brain and, together with Kety and others from the University of Pennsylvania and Goodale from Harvard, we developed the measurement of coronary blood flow with N_2O; we also could now determine the usage of substrates by the human heart. We found that the human heart prefers fatty acids, a finding which, of course, was confirmed later.

Cardiac metabolism has grown since that time and has developed to include the intricacies of molecular biology and biochemistry, but catheterization of the coronary sinus was a beginning. We concluded then that myocardial failure did not involve utilization of substrates by the heart, and later, of course, it was found that in all likelihood it is a disturbance in the mechanism of excitation and contraction coupling. I do not know whether Dr. Blalock was overjoyed at our enthusiasm in working on cardiac metabolism, but he generously let us do it, as long as we continued our studies on congenital heart disease.

Of great importance were the enthusiasm and interest of the Fellows who worked with me. Among these was Frank Spencer, who has become a prominent cardiac surgeon. There was Roy Vandam, who became the head of anesthesiology at Harvard. There were James Campbell, who is now President of the St. Luke's Presbyterian Medical Center in Chicago; Frank Grey, Jr., now in Philadelphia; and many others from abroad – from Holland, from Denmark, from Germany, from Switzerland, and from England.

When I moved to Birmingham, Alabama, catheterization was still new, and an old urologist in Birmingham informed his colleagues that he did not understand the fuss since he had done catheterization in his practice for many years.

For me, catheterization was a key to cardiac pathophysiology which led me into the field of biochemistry and biophysics of heart muscle, the development of a new discipline, that of cardiac metabolism.

In retrospect, it was a beautiful time, because all pioneering when done in the right environment is exciting as long as it does not become routine. I can only express one hope for the future: that young physicians and surgeons are obliged to spend a year in a clinical physiological laboratory. This is an advice few young physicians heed, nowadays. A most regrettable fact also is the division of purely clinical and purely investigative cardiology. This should not be, and the only way to avoid this is to have the young cardiologist and cardiac surgeon spend some time training in physiological–biochemical laboratories.

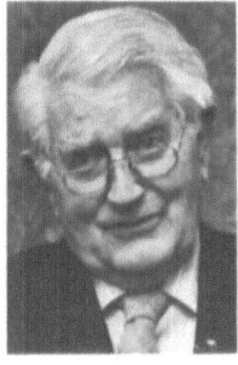

SIR JOHN McMICHAEL

Sir John McMichael, F.R.S., born in 1904, was director of the Department of Medicine of the Postgraduate Medical School of London from 1946 till 1966, and professor of medicine at the University of London. In the war years, he began right heart catheterization in London and made significant contributions toward understanding cardiac function, especially in heart failure.

Personal memories of cardiac catheterisation in Great Britain

CARDIAC OUTPUT BY GASEOUS METHODS

The problem of estimating the cardiac output had been a challenge to human physiologists in the early years of the century. Haldane's work on respiration led him to attempt to calculate the gas content of the venous blood arriving in the lungs by equilibration of the carbon dioxide content in inhaled gas mixtures. The method was practicable and some valid figures were obtained in normal man, but in the study of heart disease the application of the method involving breath-holding in dyspnoeic cardiac patients presented great difficulties. In addition, doubts were entertained as to whether gaseous equilibrium could be reached at all in the presence of pulmonary congestion and oedema. Although Meakins and associates showed that the cardiac output might be normal in cases of valvular disease, the results were regarded as unreliable, particularly by those who assumed that the cardiac output must be depressed in organic heart disease. The result was a rather defeatist attitude in the early 1930s about the possibility of estimating cardiac output in health and disease.

Direct puncture of the right ventricle had been contemplated but was generally disapproved because of the dangers.

In 1935, Tinsley Harrison published a book on 'Failure of the circulation' in which he assembled all the available data, including results from the newer acetylene method, which had been developed by Grollman, and which showed that the cardiac output might be well sustained even in the presence of some degree of heart failure. He also contrasted the clinical picture of the *hypokinetic syndrome* resulting from haemorrhagic shock with that of the breathless heart patient, and concluded that the symptoms of heart failure were not those of a low cardiac output, but were the results of congestive phenomena in the veins and the lungs, and thus he defined heart failure as a *dyskinetic syndrome*.

Up to this time, my major research had been on portal venous congestion and the regulation of portal pressure and the liver circulation. My interest in general venous congestion was a natural next step.

I began using the Grollman technique in Professor Samson Wright's laboratory at the Middlesex Hospital, but had difficulty in getting consistent results by using Grollman's modified Haldane apparatus, in which the acetylene gas was disappearing in variable amounts in the carbon dioxide absorbent. On Samson Wright's advice, I switched the method of analysis to a manometric Van Slyke machine absorbing the CO_2 in a very small volume of strong caustic soda and thus standardising the small amount of acetylene disappearing in solution. The method at once gave satisfactory and repeatable results, which I applied to normal and cardiac patients during my years in Edinburgh between 1935 and 1939 [1, 2].

We were aware of Forssmann's self-experiment, passing a ureteric catheter into his own heart, in 1929. But it needed the challenge of war-time problems of wound shock to bring Cournand and Richards to the point of using this technique to study the circulatory effects of grave injury at the Bellevue Hospital in New York. To our surprise, they showed that the catheter could be left in position for successive samplings over periods of an hour or longer, without any ill effects. Animal experimental experience had convinced me that intubation of the heart and great veins need not interfere with the rhythm of the heart. Furthermore, Forssmann's method had been used on many scores of occasions for the injection of radio-opaque solutions to clarify the interpretation of the branching X-ray shadows in the lung roots. We thus had confirmation from these many investigators in France and Portugal that the catheterisation procedure was eminently practicable.

International contacts were impossible during the War. On a visit to the Deutsche Gesellschaft für Innere Medizin in 1949, I was surprised that so little attention had been paid to the pioneering work of Forssmann. I found out his whereabouts from Professor K. Spang of Heidelberg and invited him to come to London in 1951 to participate in a film on 'Cardiac output in man' (I.C.I.). (Part of this film was shown during the meeting.) We made a fuss about him, introduced him to many eminent cardiologists and physiologists, and ensured his recognition.

EARLY CATHETER STUDIES

I carried out my first catherisation on a patient whose problem seemed incapable of solution without the procedure, and obtained samples from the right atrium, on 24 November 1942. The patient was cyanotic and also had considerable depression of oxygen in his arterial blood. He continued to have severe attacks of failure and died the following year. At the time, we thought he was shunting his venous blood through an atrial septal defect [3], but recent re-examination of the autopsy records changed my diagnosis to 'sub-acute bronchogenic cor pulmonale' or obstructive airways disease, which was only clearly defined a decade and a half later.

E. P. Sharpey-Schafer was my colleague, and we began to take advantage of this technique in investigating the then controversial action of digitalis in heart failure. But we needed normal volunteers. I went to see Sir Edward Mellanby, the Secretary of the Medical Research Council, to ask for the approval of the war-time Wound-shock Committee in seeking volunteers. Mellanby's reaction was that no committee would give its approval of such an unorthodox procedure, and the responsibility must lie with ourselves. He would have no objection, however, to my personal approach to the Friends Ambulance Unit. The first volunteer from the Quaker group for cardiac output determination, while he was simultaneously giving blood for blood transfusion, was one of the famous Quaker Cadbury family. In order to get maximum information from these volunteers, we had obtained the coopera-tion of Professor Henry Barcroft and Dr. O.G. Edholm, who were in a position to make peripheral blood flow studies simultaneously with measure-ment of the total circulation. I well remember the excitement of observing for the first time the intense vasodilatation of the forearm vessels during a post-haemorrhagic faint [4]. While the war continued with its inevitable increase in the hazards to life, volunteers were not difficult to persuade as they felt that they were contributing to the war effort by helping in these researches.

In February 1944, Sharpey-Schafer and I made our joint communications to the Physiological Society, at University College Hospital Medical School. Sir Thomas Lewis was in the Chair. He described our opening paper as 'start-ling', and at the lunch table, he shook his head hinting that we should abandon the procedure. Sir Henry Dale was at the same table, and com-mented that the total record of experience which we had assembled (394 instances) seemed to him to establish the practicability and safety of the technique, and that it was too valuable to be dropped [5]. Dale's prestige and powerful encouragement was vitally important to us at that moment.

It was already becoming clear that the diagnostic possibilities of that method were enormous, as well as the value of the technique in the study of pharmacological and therapeutic effects. We were at that time timidly limiting ourselves to right atrial catheterisation and saline manometry. But these limitations led us into erroneous interpretations. We failed to appreciate the importance of the left heart, and also of specific effects of valvular disease. British cardiology at the beginning of the war was reluctant to endorse right and left heart failure as separable syndromes. Also, the strict technical physiological principles defined by Carl Wiggers to be applied in optical pressure recording from the interior of the heart were considered impossible through a long cardiac catheter.

There was still great controversy in many quarters as to whether digitalis-induced improvement in cardiac failure was dependent on its slowing effects in atrial fibrillation, and whether the drug was effective in patients with normal rhythm. We were certainly able to show dramatic improvement in cardiac output in heart failure with sinus rhythm, but quite often the cardiac output did not improve, although the venous pressure would fall dramatically. For a time we entertained the idea that an important primary effect of digitalis might be relaxation of venous tone, causing a fall in right atrial pressure, as reduction of venous pressure by a large venesection often led to a similar increase in cardiac output. By 1946, however, we realised that digitalis effects on cardiac *work* were greater than the effect of venous pressure reduction [7]. Subsequently we realised when optical records were made that the two sides of the heart might behave differently and that relief of left ventricular failure could take place with a diminution of venous congestion in the lungs and a fall of pressure in the right heart. Improvement of left ventricular contractility need not be accompanied by improvement of output, but was manifested by maintenance of output against a higher systemic arterial pressure [8]. The concept of right and left heart failure was fully vindicated. Quite frequently, improvement in right ventricular function was also shown by increase in pulse pressure in the right ventricle, but cardiac output improvement could be frustrated by valvular incompetence or stenosis ahead.

SERVICE TO CARDIAC SURGERY AND THE NEW ERA

Soon after the war ended, Blalock developed his method of shunting blood through the lungs in children with cyanotic congenital heart disease, and the necessity for cardiac catheterisation for pre-operative diagnosis was fully justified. Other developments in cardiac surgery quickly followed, and the technique was necessary to obtain precise quantitative information about cardiac dynamics in valvular heart disease. A new era had begun in physiological assessment of heart function, to be followed by an enormous expansion of new methods of treatment and management in heart disease.

The application of modern physics to cardiac investigation has of course added even greater precision. Ultrasound has made the movement of the valves visible, and radioactive tracers enable us to see the changing patterns of coronary blood flow, at rest and on exercise, in great detail. So much information is now available that cardiac catheterisation has become less essential, as non-invasive methods can yield much detail, but nevertheless, it set a high standard of precision at the beginning of the physiological era without which the accuracy of newer developing techniques could not be checked.

Quite apart from primary diseases of the heart, the technique illuminated the circulation through the lungs and its relationship to various degrees of lung function in health and disease. It thus played its part in a great flowering of technology in the combined study of cardiac and pulmonary disorders and their interrelationships.

REFERENCES

1. McMichael J (1937) Postural changes in cardiac output and respiration in man. Q J Exp Physiol 27:55
2. McMichael J (1938) Output of heart in congestive failure. Q J Med 7:331
3. McMichael J, Foreword to Verel D, Grainger RG (1969) Cardiac catheterisation. Edinburgh: Churchill Livingstone
4. Barcroft H, Edholm OG, McMichael J, Sharpey-Schafer EP (1944) Post-haemorrhagic fainting: study by cardiac output and forearm blood flow. Lancet 1:489
5. McMichael J, Sharpey-Schafer EP (1944) Cardiac output in man by direct Fick method; effects of posture, venous pressure change, atropine and adrenaline. Br Heart J 6:33
6. McMichael J, Sharpey-Schafer EP (1944) Action of intravenous digoxin in man. Q J Med 13:123
7. Howarth S, McMichael J, Sharpey-Schafer EP (1946) Venesection in low-output heart failure. Clin Sci 6:41
8. McMichael J (1950) Observations on right ventricular pressure with digitalis. Cardiologia 15:182

PIERRE MAURICE

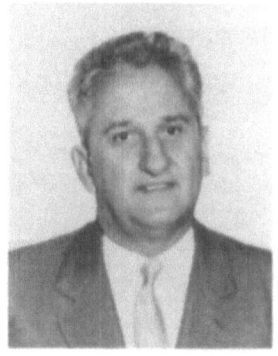

Pierre Maurice, born in 1916, was one of the chief collaborators of Dr. Lenègre, the famous Paris cardiologist. Dr. Maurice is professor of clinical cardiology and chief of the cardiac department at l'Hôpital Broussais. In 1943, as a member of Lenègre's team, he began right heart catheterization for the study of the pulmonary circulation and in 1945 he obtained the first intracardiac electrograms.

Jean Lenègre et les potentiels électriques endocavitaires

C'est en 1943 alors que j'étais son Interne que le Professeur Jean Lenègre me proposait comme sujet de thèse « l'évaluation directe des pressions intracardiaques droites chez l'homme ». L'Europe continentale en guerre et occupée n'avait alors aucune relation avec les États-Unis et la Grande-Bretagne et de ce fait nous étions totalement ignorants des travaux entrepris à New York par le Professeur Cournand et par ses collaborateurs et à Londres par le Professeur Mac Michael. Par contre nous connaissions les études angiographiques pulmonaires réalisées par cathétérisme de la veine cave supérieure par nos amis portugais et reprises en France par Ameuille et Roy.

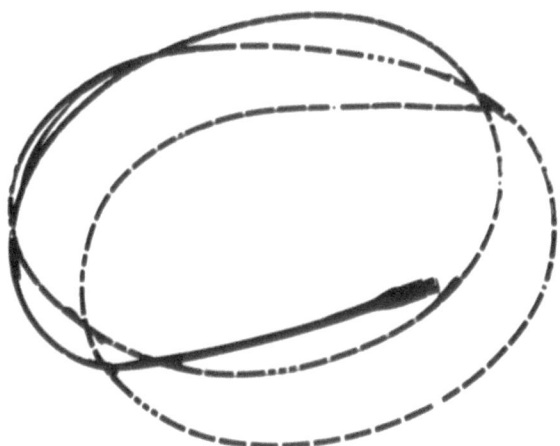

Fig. 1. Sonde urétérale en gomme n° 13 ayant permis les premiers cathétérismes en 1943.

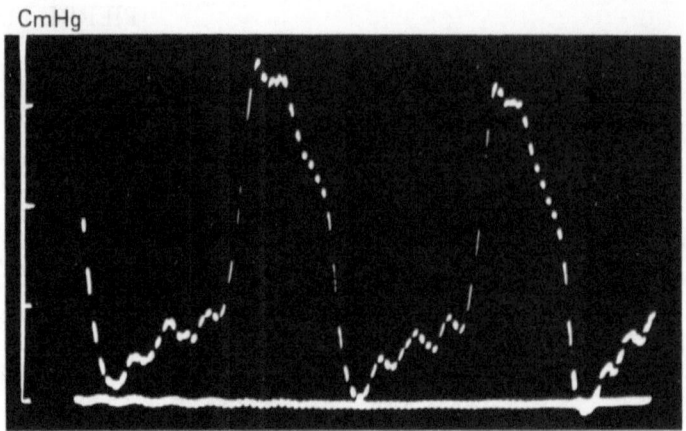

Fig. 2. Un des premiers enregistrements de courbe ventriculaire droite obtenu à l'aide d'un piézographe à condensateur variable.

Notre matériel initial, extrêmement sommaire, rigoureusemant stérile, comportait :

1° – un jeu de sondes en gomme, opaques aux rayons X, identiques aux sondes urétérales n° 13, à extrémité en sifflet et à trois orifices (Fig. 1);

2° – un trocart permettant la ponction d'une veine basilique du pli du coude puis le passage de cette sonde ;

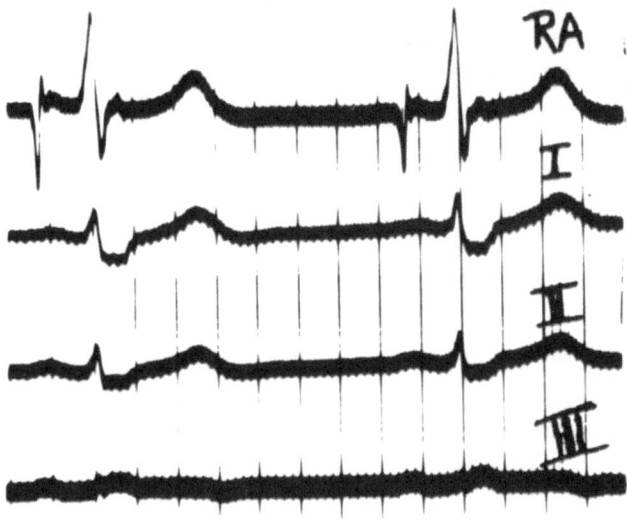

Fig. 3. Un des premiers enregistrements intra-auriculaires droits. De haut en bas : dérivation intra-auriculaire et trois dérivations standard.

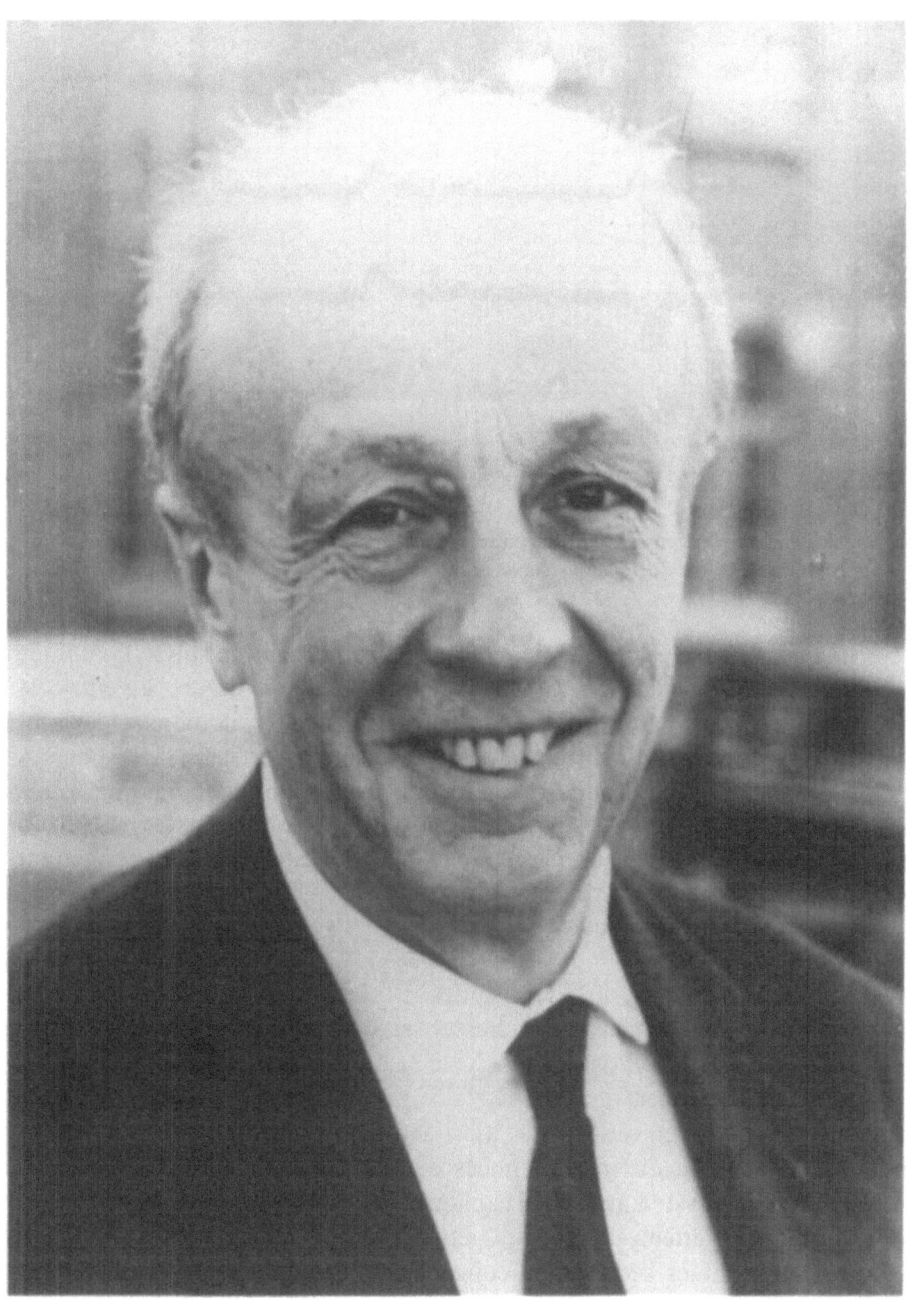

Professor Jean Lenègre, who died in 1972, is remembered, apart from the research already mentioned, for the study of progressive degeneration of the conduction system, a syndrome which now bears his name.

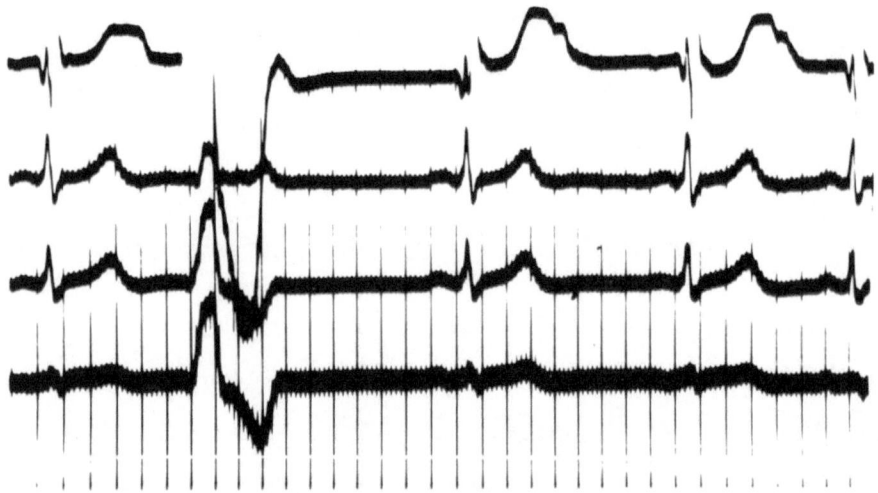

Fig. 4. Un des premiers enregistrements intraventriculaires. De haut en bas: dérivation intraventriculaire droits et trois dérivations standard.

3° – un appareil fixe et vertical de radioscopie permettant de suivre la montée du cathéter vers la veine cave supérieure, l'oreillette droite, le ventricule droit et parfois l'artère pulmonaire et obligeant à de nombreux déplacements du malade du lit d'examen à la position verticale;

4° – un manomètre de Claude relié à la sonde et rempli de citrate de soude assurant l'évaluation des pressions moyennes des diverses cavités; et un peu plus tardivement un piézographe à condensateur variable permettant d'obtenir des courbes de pressions référenciées et d'apprécier les valeurs systoliques et diastoliques.

Dès la fin de la guerre et la reprise des relations internationales, le Professeur Cournand voulut bien nous adresser les tirés à part de tous les travaux sur le cathétérisme entrepris par son école et nous aider dans nos recherches; je tiens à l'en remercier.

Avec ce matériel et cette installation sommaire le Professeur Lenègre et moi-même avons pu durant les années de guerre codifier les pressions normales moyennes systoliques et diastoliques régnant dans les cavités cardiaques droites et l'artère pulmonaire, étudier leurs variations au cours des diverses cardiopathies acquises ou congénitales, apprécier leurs modifications sous l'influence de drogues diverses telles la morphine, les digitaliques, les diurétiques.

Au cours des derniers mois de 1944 et pour la première fois au monde nous eûmes l'idée d'enregistrer les potentiels électriques intracavitaires de l'oreillette et du ventricule droits à l'aide d'une sonde constituée par un fil

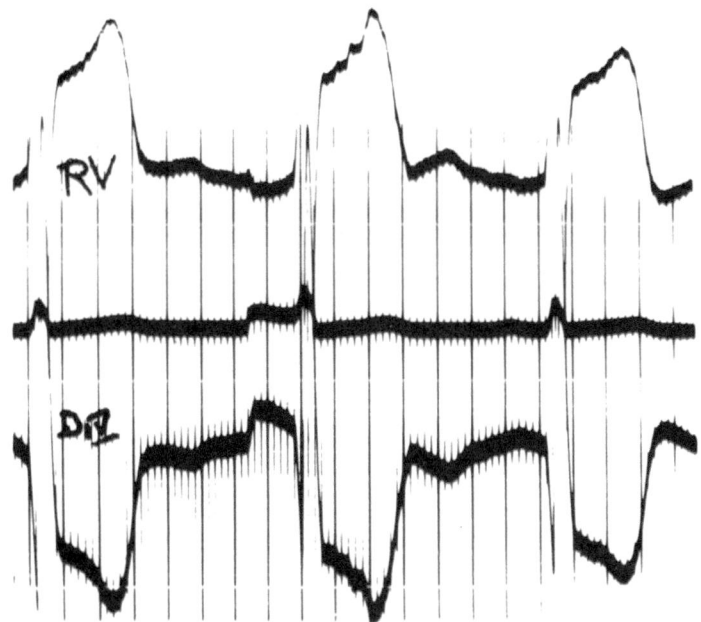

Fig. 5. Un des premiers enregistrements intraventriculaires droits.

d'or réuni d'une part à une électrode en étain et d'autre part à l'électrocardio-graphe; le fil d'or occupait la lumière d'une sonde urétérale n° 13 et l'électrode exploratrice dépassait de quelques millimètres l'enveloppe gommée. Dans la dérivation initialement employée l'électrode exploratrice était intracardiaque et l'électrode indifférente se situait à la jambe gauche. Grâce à cette méthode, par la suite largement diffusée, il nous fut possible de publier dès 1945 nos premières recherches portant sur l'origine des extra-systoles ventriculaires et des blocs de branches puis sur l'activation septale (Figs. 2–5).

Plus de trente-cinq ans se sont depuis écoulés et cependant cette période de recherche et de découverte hémodynamiques demeure dans notre carrière médicale la plus exaltante.

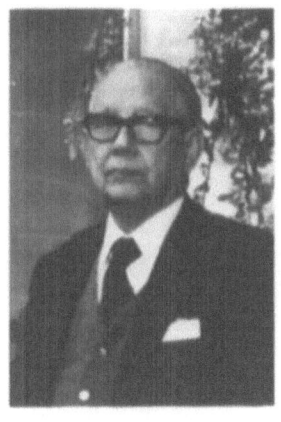

Agustin W. Castellanos, born in Cuba in 1902, was professor of pediatrics in Havana from 1932 till 1959. He is now living in Florida. In 1937 he obtained the first angiocardiograms in children with congenital heart disease. He greatly improved the technique and described his findings in congenital heart disease in numerous papers.

Personal memories of angiocardiography of cardiac malformations

As a young physician, while attending pediatric rounds dealing with patients having congenital heart disease, I always felt very unhappy when the discussant (generally the Chairman of Pediatrics) closed the case by classifying it according to Dr. Variot's nomenclature as 'congenital heart lesion with or without cyanosis and with or without murmur.' At that time, only one X-ray (anteroposterior) view was available. Later the three standard EKG leads became available.

Even at such an early date, my experience led me to believe (and state) that some day these congenital malformations could be operated upon, but the surgeon had to be given an adequate, accurate, anatomical picture. However, the consensus of opinion was against me and most persons considered this idea as only a dream, since they believed that the heart, because of it being in constant motion and, of course, full of blood, was 'taboo,' or untouchable. These criticisms did not discourage me. On the contrary, they produced the necessary stimulation for my subsequent work.

The reading of numerous articles from Europe – Forssmann, Moniz, Lopo de Carvalho and A. Lima, Ravina, Sourice and Benzaque, Reboul and Racine, Contiades, Ungar and Naullaum, Ameuille, Rinar, Desgrez and Lemoine and others – convinced me that contrast media could be used for precise anatomical diagnosis of the malformed hearts, hence enabling the surgeons to be successful in approaching the cardiac malformations. (This happened between the years 1925 and 1936.) In animal experiments (rabbits and small dogs) and in cadavers, I performed injections of Thorotrast potassium iodide and Per-Abrodil (35%). Later, the concentration of Per-Abrodil was increased to 50%.

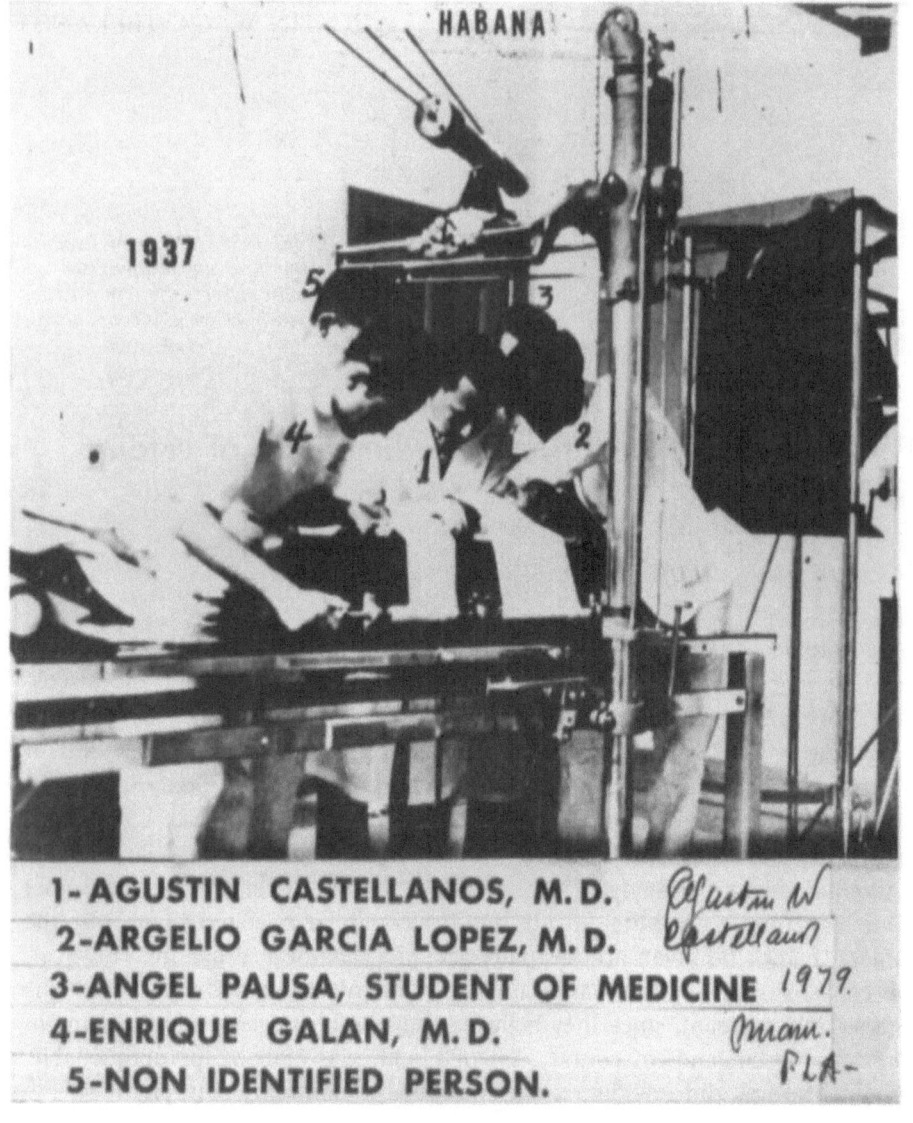

HABANA

1937

1-AGUSTIN CASTELLANOS, M.D.
2-ARGELIO GARCIA LOPEZ, M.D.
3-ANGEL PAUSA, STUDENT OF MEDICINE *1979.*
4-ENRIQUE GALAN, M.D.
5-NON IDENTIFIED PERSON.

Fig. 1. Photograph of probably the first angiocardiographic examination of man during life (1937).

I used only one film in frontal or lateral position (Fig. 1). Finally, in the meeting of the 'Sociedad de Estudios Clinicos de la Habana,' on September 1937, I presented 'The radio-opaque angiocardiography' (in cadavers and in human beings), giving the pattern of the normal cases and of the ventricular septal defect and pulmonary stenosis. I called the procedure *radio-opaque angiocardiography* because it was the radiographic visualization of the heart and the great vessels by means of contrast media.

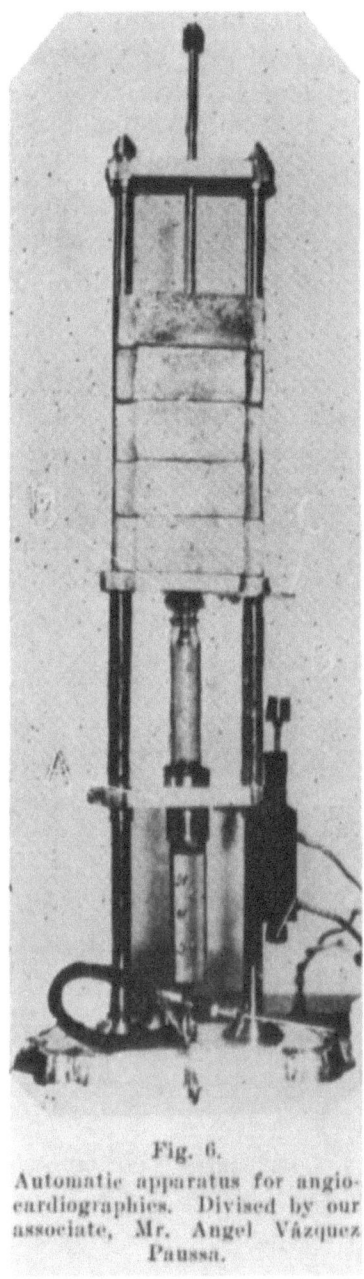

Fig. 6.
Automatic apparatus for angio-
cardiographies. Divised by our
associate, Mr. Angel Vázquez
Paussa.

Fig. 2. Automatic apparatus to perform the injection of dye (1938).

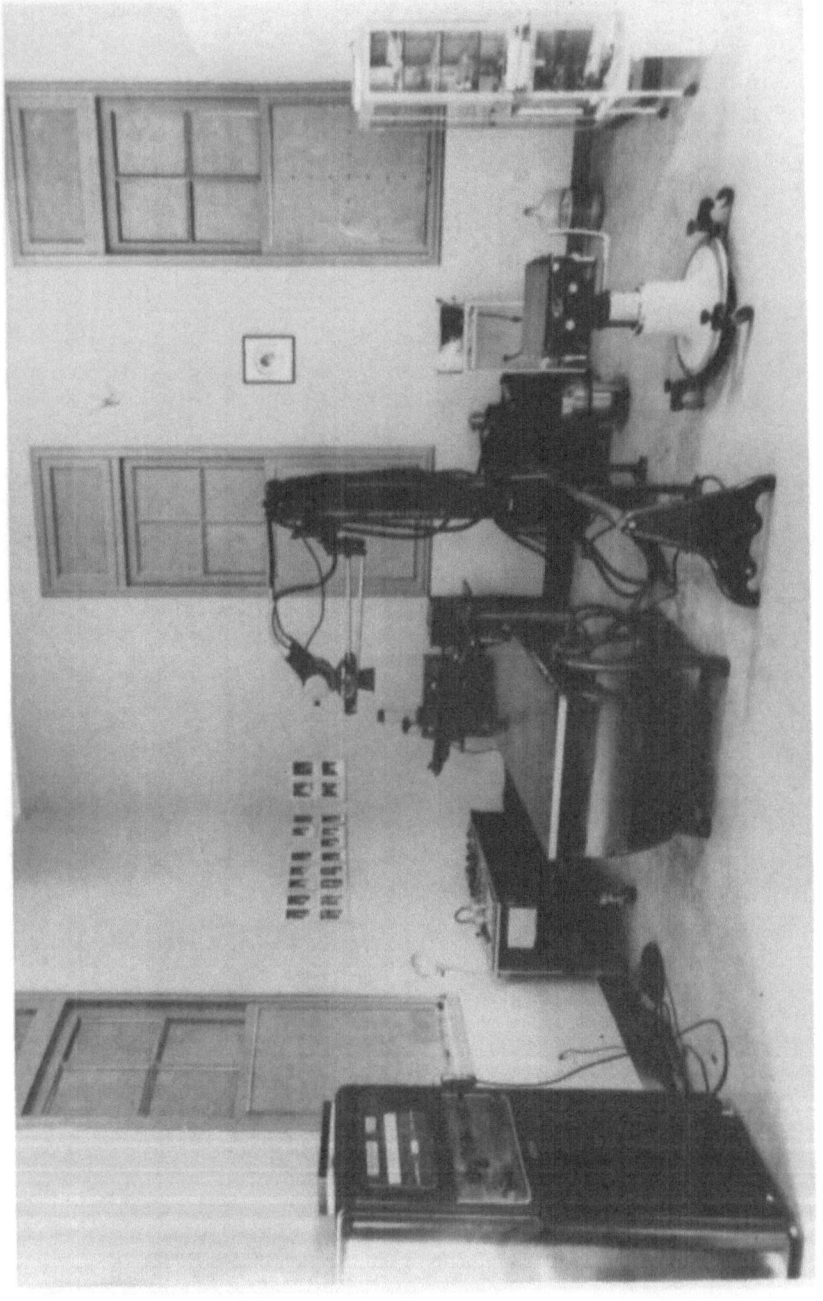

Fig. 3. Catheterization and angiocardiographic equipment (1952). In this hospital, the first cardiovascular operations were carried out.

I want to mention here a paper I have written with R. Montero and R. Pereiras, entitled 'Permanent ingurgitation of the left jugular vein in childhood. The angiocardiography in mediastinal syndromes' (*Arch. Intern. Med.* 1937). Although not well known, it nevertheless is the first article to demonstrate that the method is useful in mediastinal diseases, not only in childhood, but also in adults.

Potassium iodide 120% was utilized only in cadavers. Thorotrast was used only once without any side effect. The contrast media used at the beginning in children were Uroselectan A and Uroselectan B, but in most cases our choice was 1.5 cc per kg weight of Per-Abrodil. It had a concentration of 35%, but afterward the manufacturer at my request increased the concentration to 50%. With this concentration I obtained excellent contrast in older children.

In 1939, I originated the *retrograde* or *counter-current aortography* for the diagnosis of the patent ductus arteriosus. In 1942, this method was applied to the diagnosis of the coarctation of the aorta. In 1938, we designed an automatic apparatus (Fig. 2) to perform the injection of the dye and to do the exposure of the film at the very end of the injection of the contrast material. At that time, there were no cassette-changers.

In 1944, I. Steinberg was doing angiocardiographies on adults in New York City, taking X-ray films during the passage of the dye through the left cardiac cavities. To avoid confusion I published a paper describing the *dextro-angiocardiogram,* that is, the radio opacification of the right cardiac chambers, and the *levo-angiogram* (the visualization of the left ventricle and aorta). These terms have been accepted and widely used all over the world.

In 1953, we designed special trocars for older children and adolescents. The no. 10 trocars were manufactured by Beckton and Dickinson, enabling the injection of 40 cc of dye through a peripheral vein of the elbow in $1\frac{1}{2}$ s.

In the same year, we emphasized the value of *retrograde aortography* for the study of congenital cardiac lesions operated upon, mainly with shunts between the aorta and pulmonary artery. Moreover, I made the diagnosis of aortic insufficiency by retrograde aortography without catheterization of the aorta.

It would take too long to describe my entire work in this field in which I have worked so hard and so long. The procedures mentioned above are still being performed by many cardiologists and radiologists in spite of the well-known great advances of noninvasive techniques. Even with the latter, contrast studies still have to be performed in patients with complex anomalies where thorough knowledge of the intricate anatomy is required.

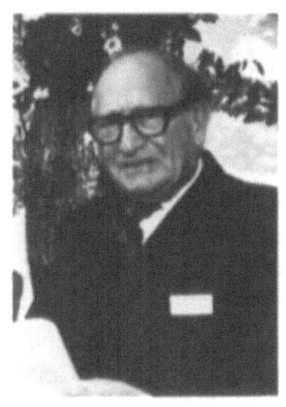

ISRAEL STEINBERG

Israel Steinberg, born 1902, was attached to Cornell University Medical School in New York since 1940, lastly as professor of radiology till 1960. Over the years, he has demonstrated the value of angiography in cardiovascular disease, especially in the diagnosis of fistulas and aneurysms of the arterial system.

Personal memories of angiocardiography

Our method of angiocardiography had its beginning when Robb and I renewed acquaintances at the evening cardiac clinic of Bellevue Hospital in 1935. We had met in Boston earlier when I had been a medical intern and he a Fellow at the Harvard service of the City Hospital. Robb's researches had been concerned with the velocity of pulmonary and peripheral blood flow, especially in stasis of the blood in the lungs during paroxymal attacks of dyspnea (cardiac asthma). His observations led him to believe that if an inert organic iodide compound could be rapidly and safely injected into the venous circulation, it would opacify the pulmonary vasculature.

Our preliminary studies in rabbits began in January 1936. Injections of 35% Diodrast, a compound in use for pyelography, was found to be well tolerated. Using amounts of Diodrast that could be safely tolerated by man and by making a special 12-gauge needle-stopcock unit with a special 12-gauge bore syringe, rapidity of injection was achieved. The pulmonary circulation of the rabbit on X-ray was not as bright as we had anticipated, so the 35% solution was boiled to half its volume and made a solution of 70% Diodrast. This was found to be well tolerated by animal and man. Using a single 14×10 inch film with the patient sitting in the erect position and having the patient make respiratory maneuvers, the right heart and pulmonary artery were visualized on 30 January 1937. Utilizing the preliminary circulation time, the left heart and aorta were visualized in man on 21 May 1937.

When a new X-ray department opened at Bellevue, permission to use the stereo-cassette unit was obtained. Working at night and making preliminary circulation time determinations, the right and left sides of the heart were readily visualized with a single injection of 70% Diodrast. When oblique or lateral views were indicated, additional injections were made. Careful clinical and laboratory studies showed that the method of cardiovascular visualization produced few untoward reactions, leading us to conclude that the method was safe and practical [1–3]. Then came studies of the heart and circulation in pulmonary and cardiovascular disease [4–9]. When the war came to the United States, Robb went into the Army and I into the Navy.

When the war ended, I returned home and resumed private practice and my appointments in medicine and radiology at the New York Hospital – Cornell Medical Center. There in 1948 began efforts to improve the roentgen technique for angiocardiography by the use of photoroentgen apparatus and a rapid film changer [10]. Later, a very satisfactory 12×12 inch roll-film magazine came into use [11, 12]. In 1949, our first publication in Europe, describing the value of angiocardiography in the differential diagnosis of mediastinal tumor and aneurysm, appeared in the *British Journal of Radiology* [13]. Two years later, Dotter and I published a book on angiocardiography [14].

Following publication of the book on angiocardiography, many diseases were investigated. These included: pericarditis (effusive and constrictive), pulmonary disease (infectious and emphysematous), and cancer of the lung. Among the subjects investigated in congenital heart disease were myxoma of the atria, pericardial tumors, reversed blood flow in ductus arteriosus, arteriovenous fistulae of the pulmonary artery, coronary arteriovenous fistulae, aortic sinus aneurysms, coarctation and pseudocoarctation of the aorta, anomalous pulmonary venous drainage, congenital absence of a pulmonary artery, agenesis of a lung, aortic sinus aneurysms, and persistent jugular lymph sacs. Aneurysms due to trauma, syphilis, and arteriosclerosis were also opacified [15].

Bilateral simultaneous arm injection of the veins enhanced angiocardiography and readily visualized the abdominal aorta and peripheral vascular system in 1958 [16, 17]. When an injector was obtained, a single arm intravenous injection made angiocardiography, abdominal arteriography, and peripheral arteriography practical [17]. Later an Elema-Schönander table was acquired and utilized for intravenous and selective study of the cardiovascular, abdominal aorta, and peripheral vascular systems [18].

REFERENCES

1. Robb GP, Steinberg I (1938) A practical method of visualizing the heart, the pulmonary circulation, and the great blood vessels in man. J Clin Invest 17:507
2. Robb GP, Steinberg I (1939) Visualization of the chambers of the heart, the pulmonary circulation, and the great blood vessels in man. Am J Roentgenol 41:1–17

3. Robb GP, Steinberg I (1940) Visualization of the chambers of the heart, the pulmonary circulation, and the great vessels in man: summary of method and results. JAMA 114:474–480
4. Steinberg I, Robb GP (1938) Mediastinal and hilar angiography in pulmonary disease. Am Rev Tuberc 38:557–69
5. Robb GP, Steinberg I (1939) Visualization of the chambers of the heart, the pulmonary circulation, and the great blood vessels in heart disease: preliminary observations. Am J Roentgenol 42:14–36
6. Robb GP, Steinberg I (1939) Visualization of the chambers of the heart and the thoracic blood vessels in pulmonary heart disease: a case study. Ann Intern Med 13:12–45
7. Steinberg I, Robb GP (1939) A visualization study of fibrothorax: identification of the cardiovascular structures. Radiology 33:291–298
8. Steinberg I, Robb GP, Roach UJ (1940) The differential diagnosis of mediastinal tumor and aortic aneurysm. NY State J Med 40:1168–1178
9. Roach UJ, Steinberg I, Robb GP (1941) Right-sided aorta with descending aorta simulating aneurysm. Arch Intern Med 67:995–1007
10. Temple HL, Steinberg I, Dotter CT (1948) Angiocardiography utilizing photoroentgen apparatus with a rapid film changer. Am J Roentgenol 60:646–649
11. Dotter CT, Steinberg I, Temple HL (1949) Automatic roentgen-ray roll-film magazine for angiocardiography and cerebral arteriography. Am J Roentgenol 62:355–458
12. Steinberg I, Dubilier W, Evans JA (1950) Twelve by twelve-inch roll film magazine for rapid serial roentgenography. Radiology 65:276–280
13. Steinberg I, Dotter CT (1949) The differentiation of mediastinal tumour and aneurysm: value of angiocardiography. Br J Radiol 22:567–572
14. Dotter CT, Steinberg I (1951) Angiocardiography. New York: Paul B. Hoeber
15. Steinberg I, Finby N, Evans JA (1959) A safe and practical intravenous method of abdominal aortography and peripheral arteriography. Am J Roentgenol 82:758–772
16. Steinberg I (1962) Bilateral simultaneous intravenous angiocardiography. Am J Roentgenol 88:38–42
17. Steinberg I, Stein HL (1964) Intravenous angiocardiography, abdominal aortography, and peripheral arteriography with single arm pressure injection. Am J Roentgenol 92:893–906
18. Steinberg I, Wescott J, Tillotson P, Halpern M (1962) Experience with an automatic table for serial peripheral vascular arteriography. Am J Roentgenol 88:1175–1182

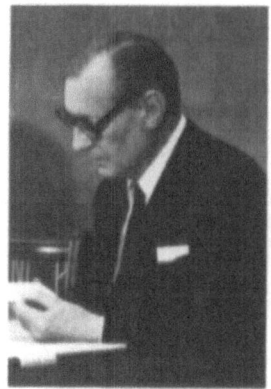

GUNNAR JÖNSSON

Gunnar Jönsson, born in 1903, trained at the Karolinska Institute in Stockholm, Sweden, and after a career elsewhere in radiology, returned to the Karolinska in 1940, where he became chief of the Department of Diagnostic Radiology from 1946 till 1969. He has made many original contributions to early angiocardiography.

Personal memories of selective angiocardiography

In the years 1947–1948, Brodén, Karnell, and I elaborated a system of methods which we called selective angiocardiography. We considered that this concept should include all examinations of the heart and the great vessels with contrast medium. The main principle was that the medium should be injected by a catheter directly into the vessel, heart chamber, or region which was to be studied or as close to it as possible in order to avoid too much dilution of the contrast medium and also to reduce superimposition of contrast-filled structures of no interest in the case. Of course, we acknowledged that the methods used were not originally invented by us. Early in 1947, Radner had shown to us that he experimentally had injected contrast medium by a catheter directly into the ascending aorta. The same year, Chavez and his colleagues published their method of direct injection into the right heart chambers.

For many reasons there was no suitable equipment available. Though Sweden was not involved in the war, there was a great lack of all technical products. As a matter of fact, our investigations were seriously delayed by this deficiency.

This was our first equipment (Fig. 1): a cassette changer made by Schönander, an injector based on a lever principle, a metal syringe, and a catheter of the Cournand type. We were very disappointed when we found that a common glass syringe burst at the first attempt. Great difficulties were involved in obtaining a metal syringe of our design with a safety device so as to avoid injection of air bubbles. At last a factory, which bored car motors, built for us a syringe suited for our purpose (Fig. 2).

69

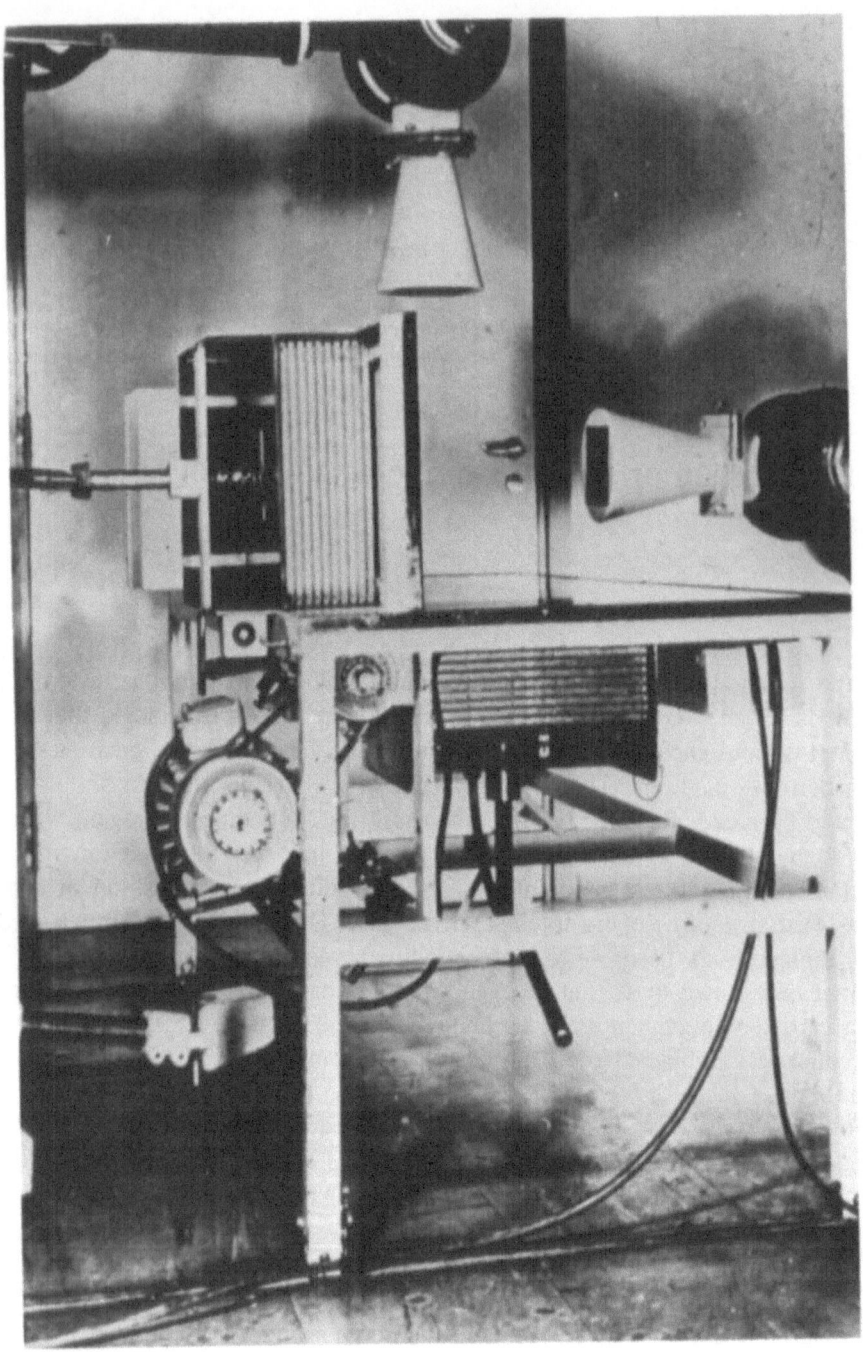

Fig. 1. First equipment.

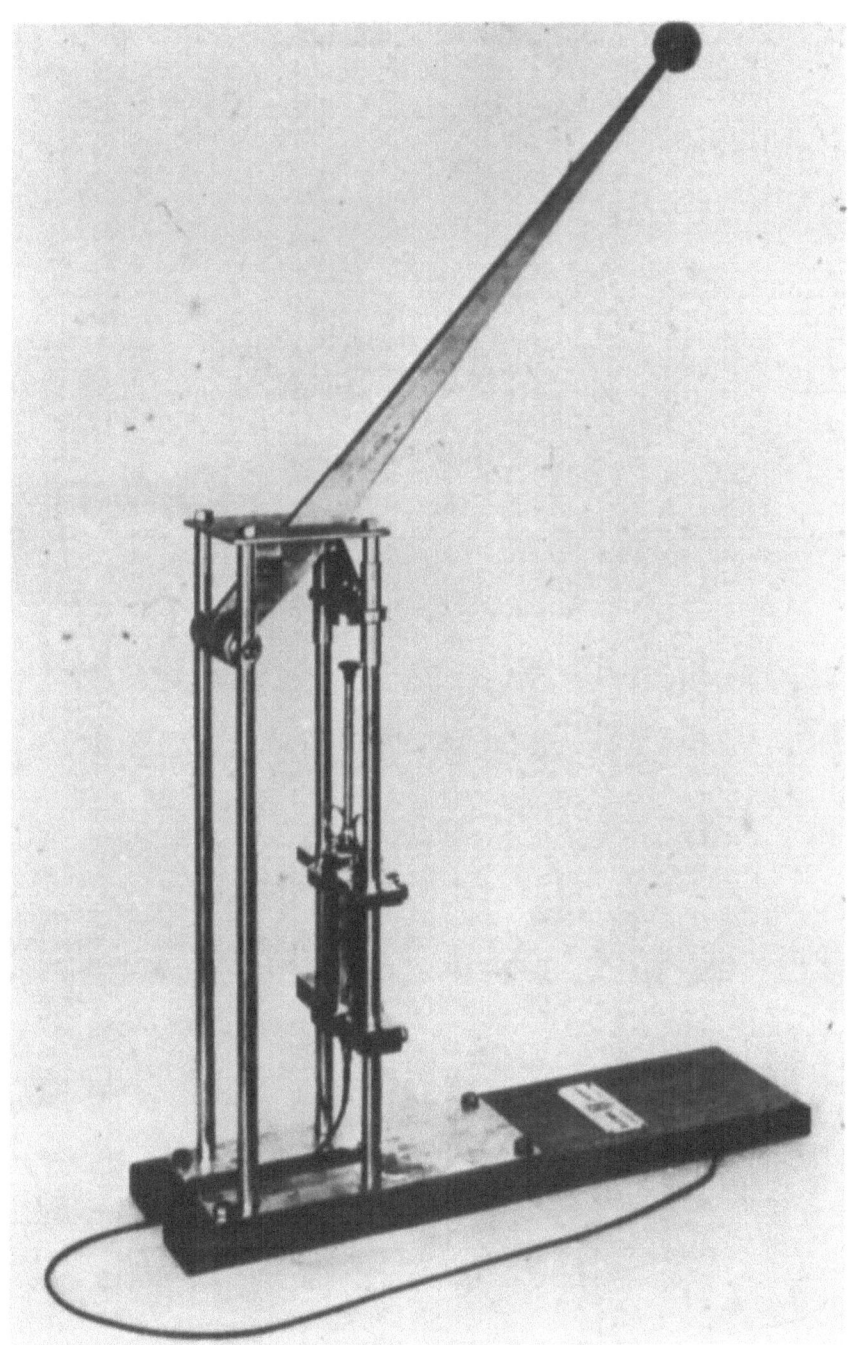

Fig. 2. Syringe for injection of contrast.

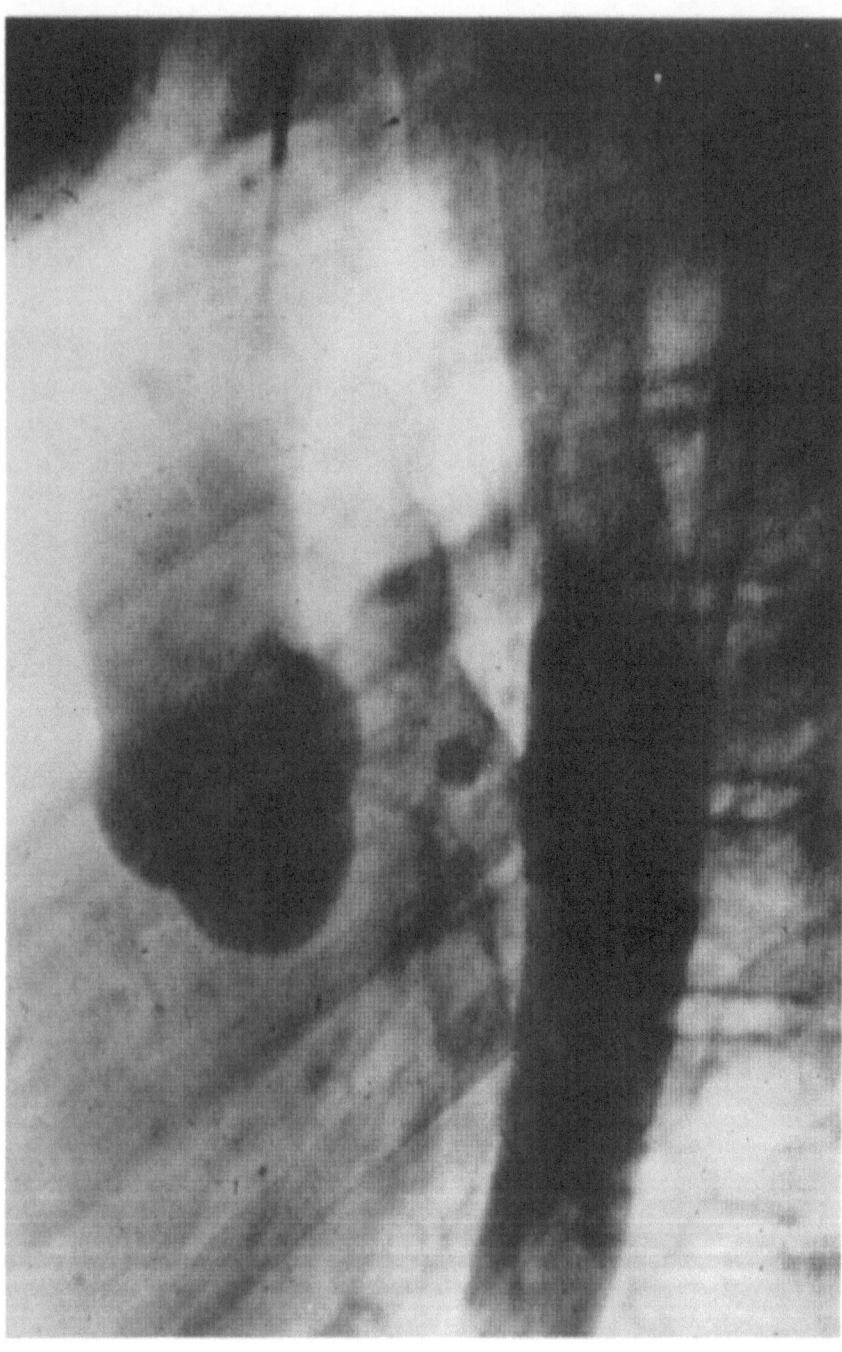

Fig. 3. Aortogram in coarctation through needle, according to Radner (left lateral view).

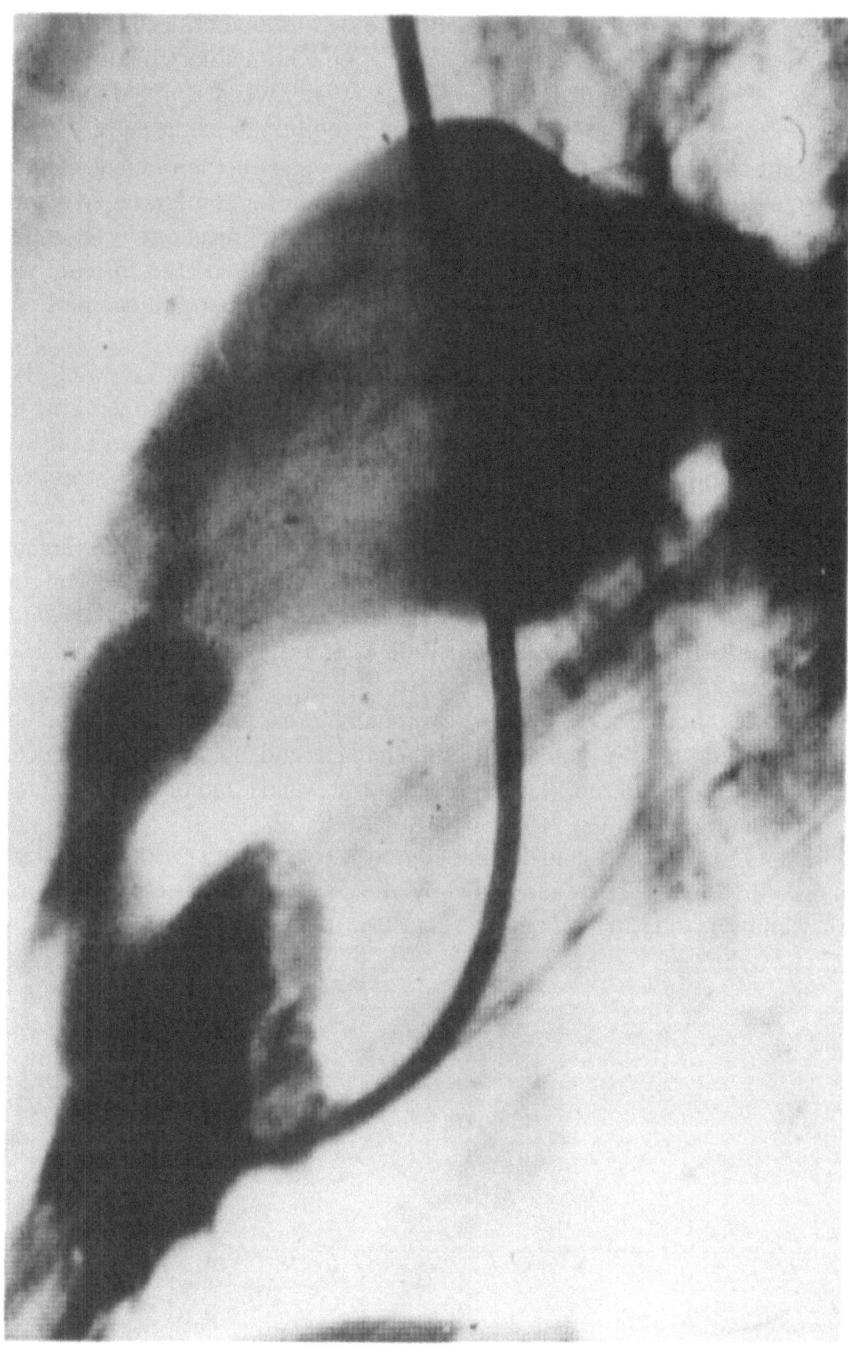

Fig. 4. Injection through catheter in right ventricle.
Pulmonary stenosis with poststenotic dilatation.

What regions did we select? Above all there was an urgent need to improve visualization of the thoracic aorta, as contrast medium injected into a vein became so extremely diluted. In November 1947, we performed our first thoracic aortography by the Radner technique, modified for clinical use (Fig. 3).

For examination of the right heart chambers, we used the original method and injected the contrast medium into a cubital vein for some time. We were not successful, however. Thus we soon changed to injection by catheter. Immediately after the cardiac catheterization was finished, the injector was connected to the catheter already in position and the angiocardiography was performed (Fig. 4).

We never punctured the heart directly through the thoracic wall. For opacification of the left atrium and left ventricle, the contrast medium, for several years, was injected into the pulmonary artery. On the basis of physiologic and anatomic observations, Arvidsson gave an extensive report on mitral valvular disease.

The aim has always been to fulfill the demands put forward by the thoracic surgeons. Thus when open-heart surgery was introduced, selective contrast examination of the left ventricle also was indicated. We had the great privilege to collaborate with a pioneer surgeon, Prof. Clarence Crafoord, and his staff from the start in 1947.

During the course of time, the equipment was gradually replaced by improved apparatus. We got a roll-film changer and an automatic injector both designed by Gidlund. Later we got thin-walled radiopaque catheters elaborated upon by Ödman at our department.

Around 1950, Kjellberg and Rudhe started their eminent work in the field of angiocardiography. They adopted fully the principle of selective visualization in children, too, and refined the methods in several ways.

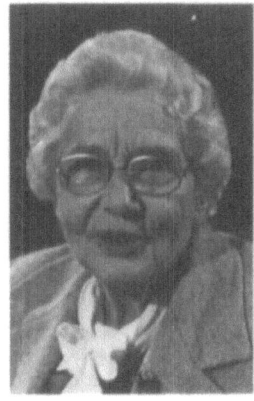

HELEN B. TAUSSIG

Helen B. Taussig, born in 1898, was in charge of the pediatric cardiac clinic at Johns Hopkins School of Medicine from 1930 till 1963 and professor of pediatrics at the institution from 1959 till 1963. In 1947, she wrote 'Congenital malformations of the heart', a classic description of congenital heart disease, its hemodynamics, and its clinical symptoms and signs, at the start of its surgical management. Together with the surgeon Dr. Alfred Blalock, she worked on the development of the Blalock–Taussig systemic-pulmonary shunt operation and did a long follow-up on its results. Today she is still active in the prevention of congenital malformations, which started with the thalidomide drama in 1962. Also, she is actively supporting women's rights, especially for abortion, and the right to die with dignity.

Personal memories of preoperative diagnostics

I have little to add to this historic report on cardiac catheterization and angiocardiography because neither of these procedures were available at the Johns Hopkins Hospital until the fall of 1945, a year after Dr. Blalock had started operating on cyanotic children.

In 1930, Dr. Edward A. Park put me in charge of the pediatric cardiac clinic. He had the foresight to install a fluoroscope in the Harriet Lane Home for Invalid Children for the use of the pediatric staff and the house officers.

Dr. Park felt strongly that new tools brought new knowledge and he urged me to use the fluoroscope. It proved to be my most useful tool. By fluoroscopy, one can see the size and the shape of the heart in different phases of respiration and one can also see the size and position of the great vessels and the vascularity of the lungs. This last-mentioned observation was extremely important because the 'Blalock-Taussig' operation was designed to increase the circulation of blood through the lungs in cyanotic patients who were dying from anoxemia.

Personal memories of postoperative infections

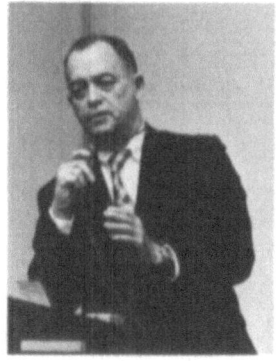

GEORGE E. BURCH

George E. Burch, born in 1910, spent his professional career in Louisiana, chiefly as professor of medicine, from 1947 till 1975. Apart from authorship of such classics as the primer of electro-cardiography, Dr. Burch has been editor of the American Heart Journal since 1959. His scientific work has ranged from the effects of hot climates on the circulation to the study of the peripheral circulation.

Historical developments in cardiology

There have been many important and exciting changes in cardiology in my lifetime. Among them the most outstanding was the introduction of antibiotics, especially the discovery of Penicillin. This advancement has essentially removed syphilitic heart disease from the roster of cardiac diseases. There is no luetic aortic valve disease and aortic aneurysm at present, and all types of syphilitic heart disease have disappeared. Prior to the antibiotic era, many patients with myocardial infarction, congestive heart failure, and other serious heart disease states died of bronchopneumonia or urinary tract infections and not of their heart disease. These infections are not complications of importance anymore. Complex cardiac and cardiovascular surgery would not be possible were it not for antibiotic agents. Infections were serious problems in the past for any type of thoracic and other surgery. The infections that complicate cardiac diseases have become less of a problem in cardiology. One can readily imagine other examples of important roles of antibiotics in cardiology and general medicine.

The advent of angiography and cardiac catheterization represents an important contribution to cardiology. The roles of Forssmann, Cournand, Castellanos, Steinberg, and others were outstanding. These contributions and the development of the cardiopulmonary bypass pump oxygenator opened the field for successful complex cardiac and cardiovascular surgery. In this regard, Alexis Carrel, John Gibbons, and many others must be remembered.

Alexis Carrel was the greatest cardiovascular surgeon in medical history to date. His contributions were outstanding. When one realizes the time in the history of medicine and medical science during which he lived, his contributions were even more remarkable. He was unbelievably dexterous and meticulous. The life of this great pioneer in cardiovascular surgery is briefly and vividly described by Edwards and Edwards. Everyone in cardiology as well as in cardiovascular surgery should read this brief biography.

It was extremely fortunate for me to have personally known Carrel, Niels Bohr, Frank Wilson, Thomas Lewis, Simon Flexner, Karl Landsteiner, Albert Claude, Tesalius, Svedberg, Fleming, and many others who contributed to the advancement of many aspects of cardiology in this century.

It is important to recognize the many contributions made to basic scientific advancements in cardiology such as occurred through electron microscopy, anticoagulant therapy, antihypertensive drugs, diet, and public health measures, to mention only a few. The development of the high-speed centrifuge, electrophoresis, chromatography, mass spectroscopy, radioelements and the tracer technic, computerized tomography and other technics, and many other developments in medicine have been explosive in nature and are tremendously important. It must be remembered that advancements in any field of medicine beneficially influence cardiology. After all, a good cardiologist is a good internist first and at all times.

There is no doubt that scientific advancements reflect the contributions of many people. Even to date the truly greatest advancement is not always easy. In the field of antibiotic therapy, Fleming surely stands out, but the contributions of the others must not be ignored. The same thought applies to the advancements which finally led to the electron microscope. Ruska and then Zworykin are prominent among these contributors. Likewise, many were involved in the development of endocrinology, antihypertensive drugs, pump oxygenators, and other advancements.

The improvements in general public health measures, such as nutrition, housing, pasteurization of milk and milk products, purification of water, mass immunization, air conditioning, heating, and clothing, have all improved the health of man enormously in the last 50 years or more of this century. The twentieth century has registered the greatest advancements in cardiology since the beginning of the history of man.

REFERENCES

Edwards WS, Edwards PD (1974) Alexis Carrel: visionary surgeon. Springfield IL: CC Thomas
Karlson KE, Dennis C, Westover D, Sanderson D (1951) Pump-oxygenator to supplant the heart and lungs for brief periods. Surgery 29:678
Marton L (1961) History of electron optics. In: Clar GL (ed) The encyclopedia of microscopy. New York: Reinhold
Nobel (1972) The man and his prizes, 3rd ed. New York: American Elsevier
Northey EH (1948) The sulfonamides and allied compounds. New York: Reinhold
Tepperman J (1973) Metabolic and endocrine physiology, an introductory text, 3rd ed. Chicago: Year Book Medical

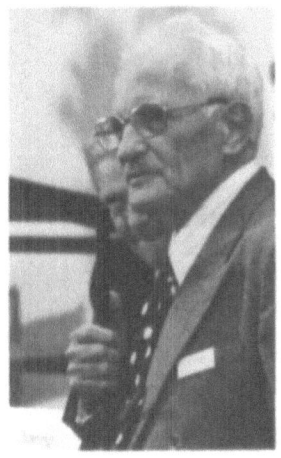

HERMAN A. SNELLEN

H..4. Snellen, born 1905, was chief of the Department of Cardiology at Leiden University from 1947 till 1972. He introduced heart catheterization in the Netherlands in 1947, and is the first President of the Einthoven Foundation, which was formed just prior to the Einthoven meeting.

The Einthoven Foundation

Since 1956, the University of Leiden has organized biennial Einthoven Lectures, which are given by pioneers in cardiology. On two occasions, the Einthoven Lecture has been replaced by an international symposium. The present meeting is the first to combine an Einthoven Lecture with a meeting in which the historical development of specific cardiological subjects (heart catheterization and angiocardiography, cardiac surgery) is reviewed in three symposia. The basic idea which can be applied to every other subject has been to divide the historical development into three stages: the earlier history, which usually will comprise the 19th and sometimes the 18th and 17th centuries; the immediate past, out of which some pioneers are still active and able to testify (it is very fortunate that so many were able to attend); and finally the present with its perspectives for the future.

To ensure the practical organization of later meetings of this type together with an Einthoven Lecture on subjects in the field of cardiology or allied disciplines, an Einthoven Foundation has been formed and duly registered in the Netherlands. This is to have a Dutch board for practical reasons, but an international advisory council. The University of Leiden participates in this Foundation and the European Society of Cardiology has agreed to cooperate.

79

PART TWO

Perspectives in cardiology

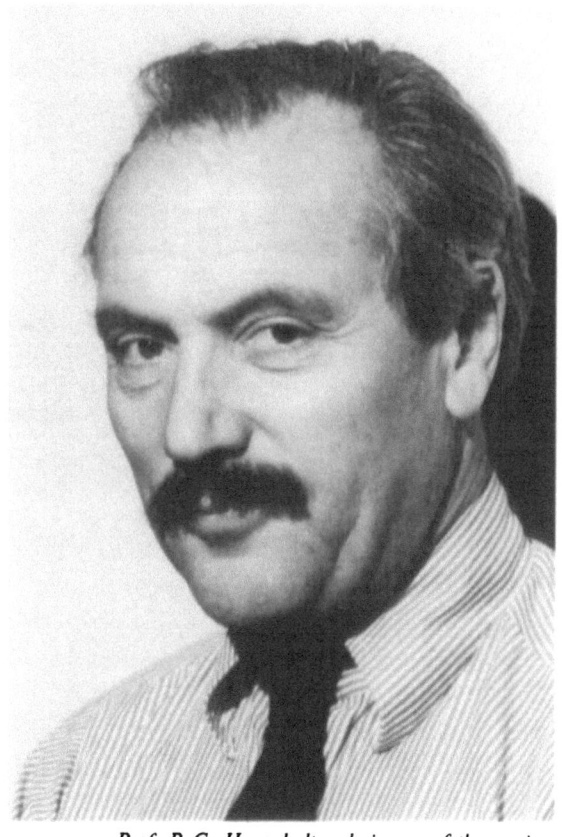

Prof. P. G. Hugenholtz, chairman of the session.

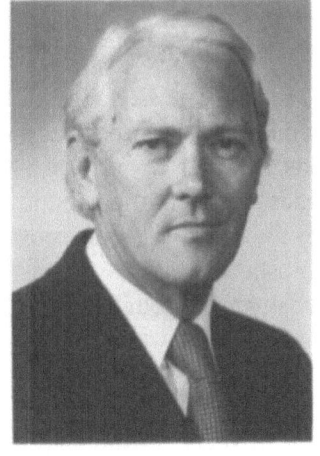

BRUCE McA. SAYERS

Bruce McA. Sayers, born in England in 1928, is a physicist who trained in Australia but returned to the Imperial College in London, where he is now professor of electrical engineering. His field of interest is biomedical engineering, as applied in experimental and clinical medicine.

Quantitation in cardiology

The cornerstones of empirical measurement in medicine are: the principle of measurement, a technology for its implementation, and two factors that relate to the interpretation of the measurement: appropriate statistical techniques to handle the inevitable variability, and knowledge about the range of normal behaviour of the variable measured. New principles of measurement in cardiology have been appearing regularly, and the technology for their implementation is certainly not far behind; but the vital factors that bear on cardiological quantitation, through analysis and interpretation, demand much closer attention than is usual, and a return to first principles is certainly justified.

The appropriate return to first principles in quantitation is a reconsideration of the relationship between measurement and interpretation in the light of recent insights and developments: the practice of measurement should certainly be fully compatible with the latest understanding of the variables being measured. So we will reconsider the fundamentals of cardiological measurement in the light of the character of the variables, as now understood. This is the more important because of the growing elaboration of cardiological measurement – which now routinely involves not only individual determinations but longitudinal observations and dynamic imaging, often of considerable technical complexity. Nevertheless, similar basic principles apply throughout.

Most cardiological variables fluctuate spontaneously and substantially. So, from the quantitative point of view, individual observations cannot justifiably be accepted as having any quantitative meaning without an accompanying specification of the uncertainty of the observation. In practice, the range of uncertainty, i.e., resolution, of simple cardiological variables is often poor and needs substantial improvement by statistical methods in order to provide a satisfactory basis for judgement in the use of modern refined therapeutic measures. Furthermore, an understanding of the relevant statistical properties is vital to the proper application of various new diagnostic methods – such as the visualisation of movements of the ventricular chambers throughout the cardiac cycle by ultrasonic or other non-invasive methods; the weight to be given to the results of this or any other measurement in assembling the complete clinical picture can only be settled with the aid of the appropriate statistics. The message of recent developments is unequivocal: cardiological measurements should, and soon will, be accompanied by a clear indication of the statistical weight that can be placed on the measurement and the likely range of uncertainty. The technology is now available to build into the next generation of instruments, from the simplest of blood pressure monitors to the most elaborate visualizing systems, all the necessary calculations and displays. Regardless of traditional practice, if quantitative as distinct from qualitative information is required from any clinical or physiological measurement, these statistical issues are inescapable.

However, the spontaneous fluctuations of cardiological variables are appreciably systematic; they exhibit longitudinal patterns. So while statistical methods are required, the statistic which applies is that of patterned signals. But the way statistical methods apply to signals exhibiting patterned – systematic – spontaneous activity does not seem to have been properly examined, or adequately put to use, in any physiological context and certainly not in cardiology. Nevertheless the matter is an important current aspect of quantitation, and an essential concomitant of the sensible and purposeful use of modern technology in medicine.

So we start our selective account of recent and future issues in quantitative cardiology with a brief examination of this crucial theoretical matter: the internal pattern structure of typical cardiological variables, the way this imposes characteristic effects on the statistical properties of the measurements, and the consequences for quantitative estimation. Then in the light of this analysis, we turn to some interesting practical problems: quantitation in electrocardiography, the analysis of records obtained by ambulatory monitoring and, finally, an area of severe quantitative difficulty – the use of closed-loop therapeutic control of the post-surgical cardiac patient.

STATISTICAL FEATURES OF PATTERN-LOADED VARIABLES

Many cardiological variables exhibit substantial spontaneous fluctuations – partly random, partly systematic. Quantitative enhancement is needed.

This applies not only to simple individual determinations but also to complete cyclic patterns; pulse pressures, for example, are variable on a beat-by-beat basis, but so are the location trajectories of the maxima of ECG thoracic surface-potential distributions. Different kinds of enhancement, still relying on the same basic concepts, are needed for some of the newer diagnostic imaging procedures that visualise the LV chamber and calculate its dynamic changes throughout the cycle; the statistical signal problems arise because of the ill-defined graduations that represent the boundaries which have to be optimally located to achieve a complete definition of the chamber and its dimensions.

All of these variables need, in one form or another, the application of the signal statistics of patterned variables. In the case of simple beat variables such as peak systolic pressure, the necessary improvement in resolution can be achieved by averaging observations at a sufficient number of successive beats. In the case of complete cyclic signals such as location trajectories of ECG maxima, or the time course of ventricular chamber dimensions throughout the cardiac cycle, the averaging is unavoidably more complex, because the set of records to be averaged must be properly synchronised to a fixed point in the individual cardiac cycle prior to averaging down the set of cyclic records at each post-reference point. But the same statistical issues arise as in the simple variable case, though in a more complicated form. And the imaging problem again compounds the complications, but draws fundamentally on the same kinds of statistical method. So the statistics of patterned signals is a generally needed development in quantitative cardiology, to parallel and sustain other technical developments.

Perhaps the most important point for the purposes of this meeting is that the development of quantitative cardiology needs such new signal statistical tools. They now exist, and are likely to influence most, if not all, cardiological measurements in the future. The central idea, though powerful, is not complex if approached through a simple kind of application – improving the resolution of a simple variable such as peak systolic pressure in the systemic arterial system. (For an ambulatory subject, a stable record might exhibit a resolution of 20 mmHg even for 1-min averaged pressure observations, a figure that is much too large to be acceptable for such studies.) The method is as usual, to draw upon repeated observations.

The important question is: how much new information can be brought in by making repeat observations? The more predictable the new data, the less value it has to improve the picture we already have. Accordingly, the appropriate statistical descriptor for our purpose is the average extent to which new data can be predicted from previous data, i.e., the serial correlation sequence of the set of data, which expresses the extent of relationships, on average, between observations spaced by differing times. If sequential observations are subject to systematic pattern effects then, to some extent, later observations will indeed be predictable from earlier ones, and new observations will therefore contribute little independent information. The more independent data can be used, the less variable and more useful the averaged value will be. So the key measure is the effective number of independent observations in a given sample, from the variability viewpoint; but this is precisely the measure that can be described as the number of statistical degrees of freedom in the sample. Divided by the number of actual observations, this yields a useful measure, the number of degrees of freedom per individual observation point (df/pt). For fully independent data, this measure approximates unity; typical values for cardiological variables of all types lie between 1/30th to about 1/5th of this, due to the strong patterning in the data, and these figures have serious consequences for clinical measurement. Such figures apply to derived measures such as peak systolic arterial blood pressure (or the corresponding LV variable as illustrated in Fig. 1) LV (dp/dt) max, the various intracycle

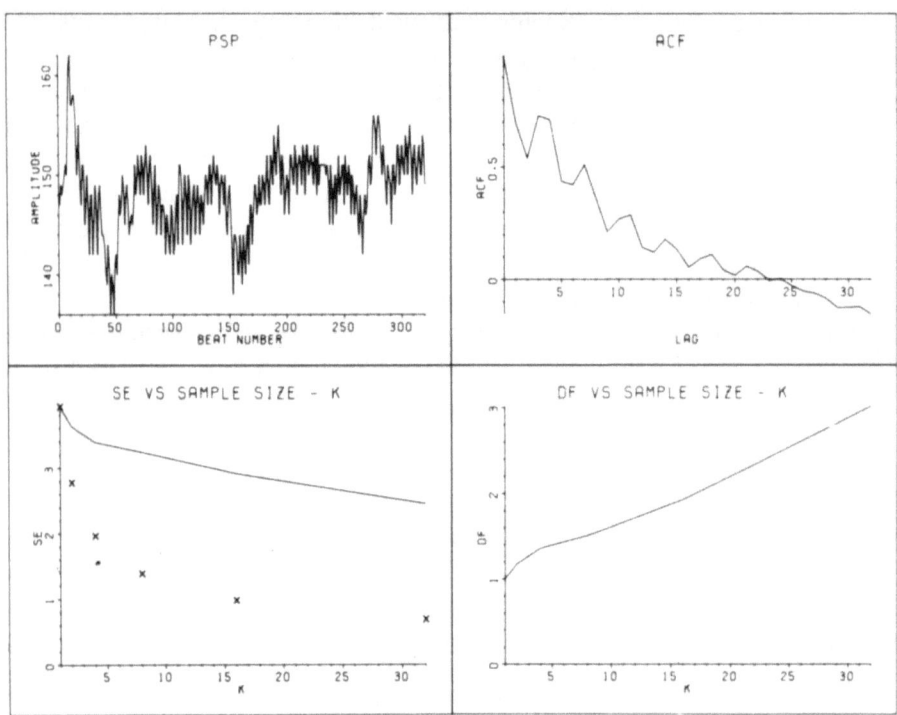

Fig. 1. A sequence of intra-ventricular peak systolic pressures, and the corresponding correlational structure of the data. The standard error SE of the mean of a sequence (size k) against k is shown for the real data, together with the curve for the same data fully randomised prior to forming sequences of size k. The effect of systematic structure in the raw data sequence is evidenced by the slower reduction of SE with size of the sequence; this is matched by the small rate of rise of the total df in the sequence.

intervals, as well as to the cyclic changes of LV dimensions and volume and of similar variables. Typical sources of systematic variation in a simple variable such as arterial blood pressure are respiratory activity, and the fluctuations of vasomotor mediation that originate in the dynamic regulating functions of the blood pressure system and of the first-line thermoregulatory system.

Two questions occur to us in this approach: how much improvement, if any, is required in the measurement we are making, and how many observations must be averaged to produce this result? We can describe the dispersion of the data by its standard deviation, and if the data is Gaussian (it may be), then we can use 2(SD) to specify the resolution (the minimum change that can be treated as significant). Averaging over a data sample with df degrees of freedom produces a mean with a dispersion (standard error, SE) given by $SD/df)^{\frac{1}{2}}$ and a resolution of 2(SE). So the necessary improvement fixes the required df. From the correlational structure of the data we can estimate the df/pt, so we can then decide on the necessary number of observations to use. Often this number is disturbingly large for realistic improvements in resolution. The sometimes very slow reduction in SE with size of data sample is illustrated for LV peak systolic pressure in Figure 1; the strong correlation effects have a major influence on the statistics.

Summarising this application then, a sequence of n observations that are appreciably correlated in this way will comprise many fewer than n independent numbers, because later observations are, on average, predictable from earlier ones. The total number of independent observations corresponds approximately to the statistical concept of degrees of freedom, df; dividing df by the number of data points (n) leads to the useful measure: degrees of freedom per point (df/pt). Typically, cardiological data generate df/pt figures between 0.03 and 0.15.

The relevant formula can be deduced in various ways; the df/pt measure for a k-point sample of observations drawn from a record with serial correlation coefficients $R_1 R_2 R_3 . : . R_{k-1}$ is given by:

$$df/\text{pt} = \frac{k}{k + 2 \sum_j (k-j) R_j} \qquad (\text{for } j = 1, k-1)$$

and is itself a statistical variable, since the various R coefficients must be estimated from the experimental data; at least $10\,k$ points are needed to make the R estimates at least potentially reasonable.

In practice, the df/pt measure is a non-linear function of sample size (Fig. 1). Further, it alters with the nature and magnitude of the underlying processes contributing to the signal concerned. Hence there are two practical ways of utilising the information it presents. First, given the observed SD of

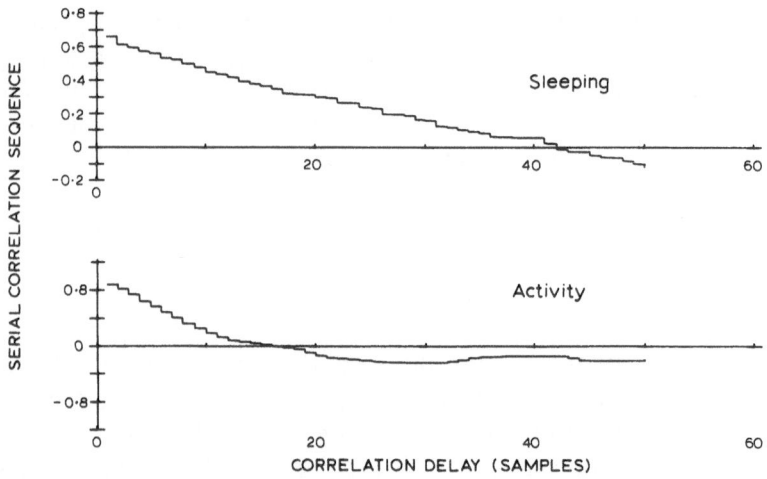

Fig. 2. Typical correlational structure of ambulatory intra-arterial blood pressure records (mean BP T3030), for the sleeping period and for daytime records. The daytime (activity) records lead to a *df*/pt estimate of 0.18; for the sleeping records this falls to 0.06. Delay samples are in units of 0.8 min.

the data, and the required SE, the necessary *df* can be calculated; from the *df*/pt data for various sample sizes, the sample size needed to achieve the required *df* can be established. This approach assumes sequential data, such as from successive beats, but in any case organised exactly like the data from which the correlational estimates were made. On the other hand, if data samples could be so selected as to be, on average, independent, then the sample size needed would exactly equal the *df* (a much more efficient approach).

The necessary selection can be based on the observed correlational structure of the data (Fig. 2), focussing on the spacing of samples that generates zero value coefficients. Observations at an average spacing of 15 basic data intervals, as in Figure 2 for the activity records, or 12 min, will be essentially uncorrelated and ensure efficient and useful quantitation. Note that the choice of sampling protocol must be adapted to suit the character of the signal; compare the two curves of Figure 2. The various operations involved in this approach lend themselves readily to microprocessor implementation, and indeed a general purpose statistical interface unit for cardiological measurements is already available; the next generation of cardiological instruments should certainly reflect these developments.

The second way of using this *df*/pt information is in comparing two sets of measurements made at different times in an individual patient. To the extent that the data is Gaussianly distributed with a small figure for *df*/pt, the *df* for any reasonably sized sample will be small, and this is the figure to be used in a *t*-test statistical comparison of samples.

In short, the fundamentals of quantitative cardiological measurement, even at the simplest level, depend greatly on statistical properties of the variable which in turn, as now understood, are greatly influenced by the internal pattern structure of the sequential values taken up by the variable. The same kind of effects dictate the sensible use of the advanced technological innovations now being introduced into diagnostic cardiology.

ASSESSING MINIMUM AND MAXIMUM REQUIREMENTS FOR CARDIOLOGICAL MEASUREMENT

An important task for the would-be measurer of cardiological or other physiological variables is to ensure, first, a reasonable technical match between his technique and equipment of measurement and the variable to be measured and, second, that the interpretation does not impose an unreasonable weight on the resolution and stability of the measurement. When substantial variability exists in the variable, the appropriate questions can only be answered statistically, based on an empirical study of sufficient scale to yield fully representative descriptions of both normal and pathological records.

Such a study does not appear to have been undertaken in most variables of clinical interest, although it is necessary. In consequence, a pilot project was initiated by the Committee for Medical Research of the European Community; intra-arterial BP was used as the pilot variable. The target is the preparation of a guideline document that would, as a result of an examination of the statistical findings, allow the minimum and maximum requirements to be specified for measurement of this physiological variable, as well as the appropriate resolution, requirement for enhancement, desirable protocols for repeated observations, quantitative consequence of technological inadequacies of instrumentation, and the implications for interpretation and use of the results.

The main statistical information usually needed is: probability density (estimated by histogram) and its mean and standard deviation, serial dependence of the data as described by their serial correlation, and degrees of freedom per observation point: this information being required for each variable normally derived from the original measurement and being determined again for the typically pre-processed variable. Each derived variable is further described by certain individual features – for example, the statistics for the compensatory response in PSP, say, following a single abnormally low or high value. (These various measures were determined for a range of subjects studied under laboratory or ambulatory conditions, but it is recognised that many subjects, and patients, must be investigated.)

The effect of specifiable technical limitations on the measurement can readily be investigated by a computer simulation that operates on the unrestricted observations. Implications for design and interpretation then follow because the quantitative influence of specific instrumental design features on the variable can be determined. Also, for example, suitable design simplifications can be selected objectively for purposes such as screening, field surveys and other tasks in which relaxation of requirements is possible.

In cardiology, perhaps the most urgent guideline recommendations are those needed for the intra-cardiac dimension variable and its rate of change, and for the dynamic maps of thoracic surface cardiac potential (and particularly for inferred epicardial potentials) now being more widely utilized. The latter case is a classic situation in which a variety of ad hoc standards and procedures could easily proliferate, unless objective decisions can be agreed on the basis of the known properties of the (multi-dimensional) variable, again as assessed in sufficiently large groups of normal subjects and pathological cases.

AMBULATORY MONITORING OF CARDIOLOGICAL VARIABLES

Some recent attempts to obtain, inter alia, base-line information in cardiology utilise long-period ambulatory monitoring of blood pressure and ECG in the unconstrained subject. These attempts have produced several interesting problems of quantitation which complicate the necessary task of comparing subject groups studied in separate clinical centres, and which may comprise physiologically different populations for genetic, nutritional, environmental, or social reasons. This type of work is a variety of epidemiology; the epidemiological role is to establish base-lines for behaviour of the variable concerned in the normal population, taking account of the inter-subject variability that originates in many causes, some biological, some social. The quantitative task of signal description must be divided to handle the various difficulties that arise. First, there is a substantial non-stationarity (time variation of the short-term statistics of the signal) due to patterns of activity. Second, there are both intra-subject and inter-subject differences in the duration of sleeping periods. These patterns complicate the task of describing individual records or identifying common features that will characterise a specific group of patients. Both difficulties are met in the analysis of intra-arterial blood pressure recordings, and they are sufficiently severe to dominate the quantitative description of this variable, unless prevented.

For any group of patients, the two tasks are: to characterise the ambulatory blood pressure records during activity, and separately during sleep, despite the presence of non-stationarity; and then to provide a description of the 24-h

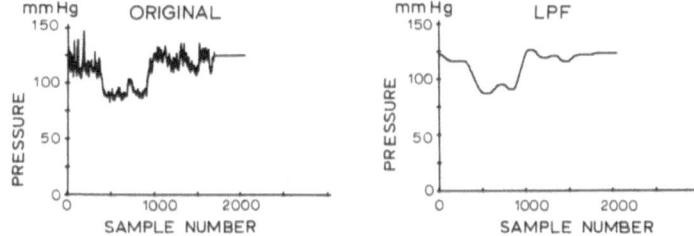

Fig. 3. Intra-arterial mean blood pressure data (24-h record T3030) from an ambulatory subject. On the left, the original data, and on the right, the low-pass filtered signal ready for circadian pattern analysis (by a Fourier phase spectral method, for example).

pattern, despite the differing rest-period durations on different days or in different subjects (Fig. 3).

The two problems can be handled in the following way. Non-stationarity in blood pressure has been identified as primarily affecting the short-term mean. Accordingly it is possible to divide the record into convenient segments, fit a trend line which can be described by its slope and duration (histograms of these variables can be employed to produce an overall picture of these sporadic trends), followed by trend removal – leaving presumably stationary records for the daytime period, and separately for the night-time

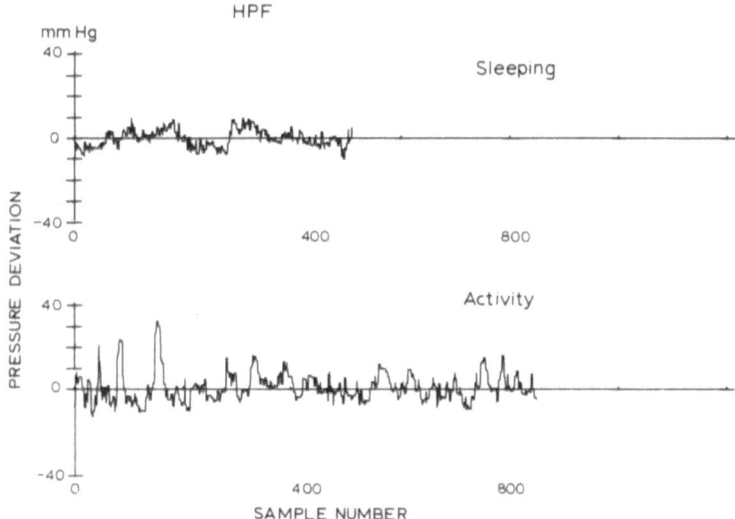

Fig. 4. Ambulatory data (0.8-min sampling interval; mean BP T3030) extracted from the record of Figure 3 by removing the circadian pattern and segmenting in two parts, with trend line removal to eliminate non-stationarity where necessary. The records are thus in a form suitable for detailed analysis (by first-order statistics, correlational structure analysis, and feature analysis, for example).

period. Ensembles of records can therefore be assembled representing typical behaviour of each of a number of subjects in the daytime or activity period (Fig. 4), and a separate ensemble formed from the corresponding records during the sleeping or resting period; these are amenable to description in standard statistical terms, subject to the influence of systematic pattern effects in the records. Since some subjects exhibit strong oscillations at all times and others show long-period recurrent fluctuations during sleep, pattern statistics are also needed in the longitudinal description of such records amongst the ensemble.

The 24-h patterns also need to be characterised. There are two approaches. One is to standardise the duration of the sleep period with a constant level interpretation in the middle of the period, and describe the resulting pattern in terms of the Fourier phase spectrum of the low-order harmonics. The other is to identify the main features of the 24-h record (the night-time decrease in mean pressure, and the matitudinal recruitment to daytime levels, say) and describe these individually, for example by curve fitting a trend line and so separating the feature into the systematic change and the deviation about it.

Either approach permits the compact description and comparison of ensembles of records in respect of each of the several main features which can be discerned. All records are put on a common basis, so that their differences are not due to inconsequential causes which otherwise create substantial changes in the signal and its quantitative description.

ELECTRO-CARDIOGRAPHIC QUANTITATION

Obtaining numbers from electro-cardiograms used to be merely a matter of measuring a few time intervals, polarities, average magnitudes, rates of change, and vector directions. But since it is now suspected that linear and vector electro-cardiography is, for technical reasons, incapable of representing the whole available cardiac potential information, a new dimension of problem has emerged – how to obtain quantitative measures from spatio-temporal patterns: the total surface distributions of thoracic potential, altering throughout the cardiac cycle. Surface mapping is an interesting pictorial portrayal of the total superficially accessible activity, but it does not lead directly to compact quantitative descriptions.

In these circumstances, one is forced back to the quantitation of important pre-selected features of the spatio-temporal patterns. Notable features of these records are the movements of potential extremes throughout the cardiac cycle, and their fluctuating intensity. Movements can be represented by plotting their trajectories throughout the cycle, and the intensity of activity at each instant can be assessed in terms of the spatial rates of change of potential away from local maxima. Trajectories can be approached either in two-dimensional terms or as two, possibly independent, one-dimensional variables corresponding to the two spatial axes of the surface. But either way, identifying standard patterns and recognising abnormalities in individual beats or distinguishing between patients cannot be achieved without a consideration of the spontaneous variability of these trajectories. There is a noticeable beat variation in the trajectory and, accordingly, a need to average trajectories in sequential beats.

This raises the question: how much improvement is needed, and how much is achievable? This again raises the issue of the number of degrees of freedom per beat for each point on the trajectory throughout the cardiac cycle. Since there is a systematic beat-by-beat change in the trajectory, due to the influence of underlying physiological mechanisms, it follows that exactly the same kind of questions apply as discussed earlier for one-dimensional variables. But given the average trajectory and the known variability, the possi-

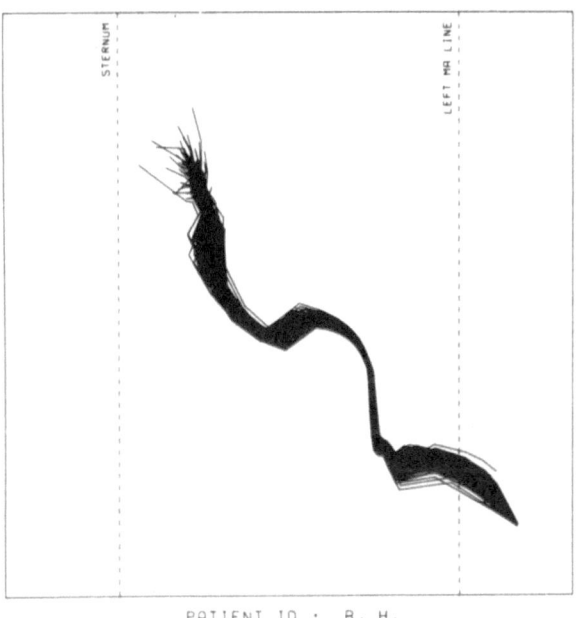

PATIENT ID : B. H.

Fig. 5. Trajectories, during 100 sequential QRS complexes, of the instantaneous position of the positive maximum of cardiac electrical potential on the anterior thorax. Each trajectory is shown for 64 ms at a sampling interval of 2 ms. Dashed lines show the sternal and left mid-axillary location. Vertically, the area shown covers approximately the region between the second intrasternal space down to about 1 cm above the umbilicus in the cardiographically normal 25-year-old man. Movement is from top left to bottom right (reached at about the peak of the R wave); the maximum shown is subsequently followed down by a secondary maximum almost immediately.

93

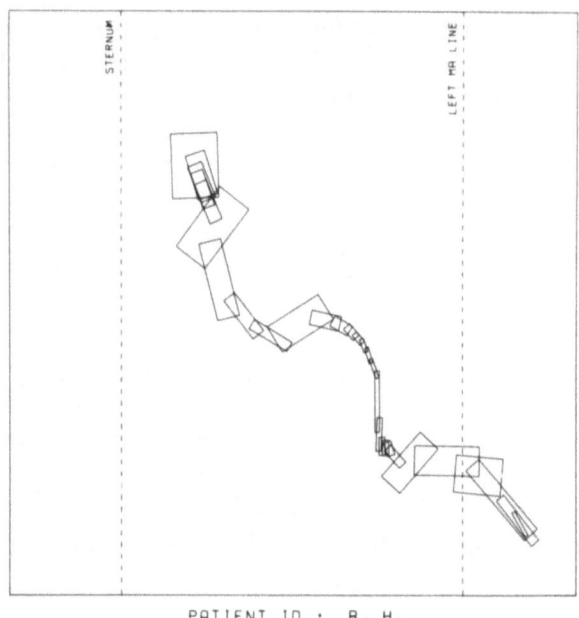

Fig. 6. Box frames at each instant showing the variability of trajectory locations at the corresponding instants in each cardiac cycle for the data shown in Figure 5. The frames are oriented along the ensemble mean direction of movement at each instant (timings referred to the R-wave peak in V_5).

bility exists of recognising individual abnormal beats and of identifying changes and trends in this specific feature of the spatio-temporal pattern, utilising well-proven statistical techniques combined with the special procedures due to the presence of patterns in sequential versions of the feature.

Figure 5 shows the extent of variability in the successive trajectories from that part of the QRS for which the major maximum of potential sweeps down from a high near-sternal position towards and beyond a low left mid-axillary position. Locations have been calculated at a 2 ms intervals for 34 instants in the cardiac cycle referring, in this case, each cycle to the instant of the R-wave peak in lead V_5. (The movement of this maximum from top left to bottom right, reached at about the time of the R-wave peak, is normally followed by the passage of a second potential maximum that again traverses part of a similar pathway before diminishing to low level.)

A clearer idea of the variability is given in the box-frame picture (Fig. 6) for the same data; the range of positional variation is shown for each of the 34 instants shown in Figure 5, orienting the frame along the ensemble mean direction at each instant.

The variability is only acceptably small for a small part of the cycle; elsewhere it needs improvement, for example, by coherent averaging. If a

94

factor of 3 improvement in the direction of the movement was required – a realistic target – a data set of sequential values exhibiting 9 df would be needed. Calculating the serial correlational values, and using the formula quoted above, leads to an estimate of df/pt for a 9-point sequence, giving a total df of 4 and an RMS improvement in position, by coherent averaging, of $\sqrt{4} = 2$. In fact, about 24 beats need to be averaged (at 0.38 df/pt) to achieve the factor of 3 improvement.

This is one example of quantitation by feature analysis which will need to be much more generally applied in the future, for instance in inferred epicardial potential maps, and thoracic surface distributions in phono-cardiography. Other kinds of feature would be appropriate for ultrasonic images of the cardiac chamber and, as discussed below, others again in the domain of the automated dynamic regulation of patients.

TREND ANALYSIS AND CLOSED–LOOP CONTROL

When a patient's physiological variables change to an appreciable extent and at a significant rate, a therapeutic response may be appropriate. This may be of particular significance in cardiology because of the time-scale over which severe changes may occur – particularly in the post-surgical patient. Trend analysis aims to recognise potentially important alterations in patient condition by identifying the occurrences of progressive changes in relevant variables. Successful identification of a trend is the occasion for a further, unspecified, decision about a therapeutic response. Closed-loop control is, in a sense, the logical extension of the recognition that therapeutic steps are needed: it actually makes the appropriate response – which is feasible only if the physiological system is sufficiently well understood that a suitable response actually is already known and if the intensity of response required can be calculated from the current state of the patient.

It the rates of change are rapid, the measurements on the patient must be regularly updated and the physiological response dynamics also need to be assessed, and used in designing and operating any closed-loop control system. One of the earliest systems of this type, perhaps the first in routine clinical use, was that designed to stabilise the state of cardiac patients following open-heart surgery, introduced by Kirklin and Sheppard. This recognises the four main determinants of left-ventricular function (afterload, myocardial contractility, preload, and heart rate) and aims to control the left ventricle by regulating the first, or perhaps the first two, of these.

In order to make possible the closed-loop control of, for example, afterload, the quantitative dynamics of the mean arterial pressure response to infusion of a suitable hypotensive agent (e.g., the vasodilator sodium nitroprusside) must be determined. Empirical evidence shows that this physiological system is linear (or at least piecewise linear), so the system dynamics, expressed in the form of the 'impulse response', can be achieved by cross-correlating the simultaneous infusion rate and mean arterial pressure signals, whilst modulating the infusion rate of the drug with a pseudo-random binary pattern. However, the stimulated response is superimposed on a spontaneously fluctuating background so, again, it is necessary to consider the statistics of the situation, and perhaps to identify those features of the estimated response that are sufficiently stable to be used in practice (Fig. 7).

The impulse response calculated in this way does often exhibit substantial variability of morphology and scale due to background activity. However, the characteristics of the spontaneous fluctuations can be determined and examples of the typical response are available, so it is feasible to carry out an empirical analysis to identify those features of the response that reliably indicate their presence against the background activity. The necessary analysis starts with a numerical simulation of a very large ensemble of records, each having the character exhibited by the actual recordings of spontaneous mean arterial blood pressure obtained from representative patients. The different members of the ensemble are obtained by the technical device of reconstituting each from the average Fourier amplitude spectrum of the actual recording (randomising within the observed range for each individual record) and a fully randomised phase spectrum. To each such simulated record (the left-hand set

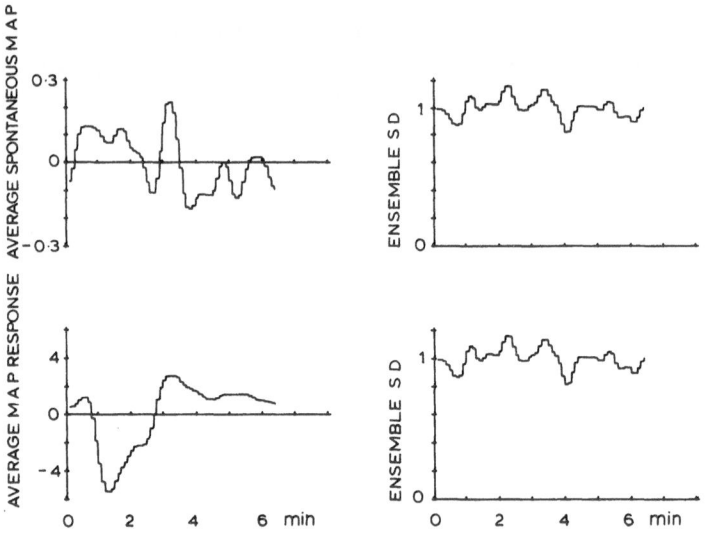

Fig. 7. Ensemble mean and SD of repeated estimates of mean arterial pressure impulse response to a bolus infusion of vasodilating agent; comparative results for spontaneous records are also shown.

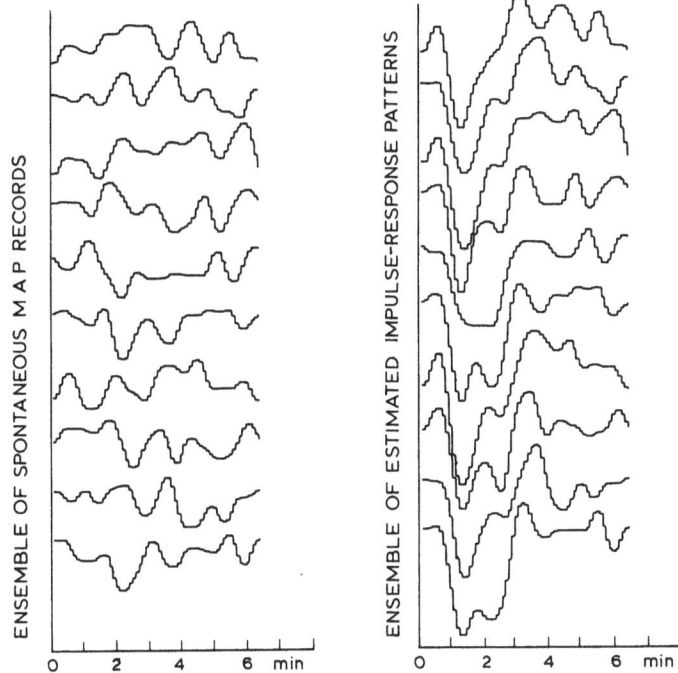

Fig. 8. Procedure for investigating the feature variability of the MAP impulse response as a result of variations of the spontaneous MAP background to which the response is added. On the left, an array of phase-randomised records obtained from an example of real spontaneous data; on the right, the result of adding to each the standard impulse-response pattern. Feature analysis identifies those features of the response that can reliably be expected to sustain through the range of spontaneous interference shown.

in Fig. 8), an actual typical response pattern is added; the result simulates a typical product of the whole practical operation of impulse-response estimation (see Fig. 8, right-hand set of curves). A statistical analysis of each individual pattern feature then completes the task.

In the case of the vaso-active response, the one stable feature is the time to reach maximum effect of an (conceptual) impulse infusion; as it happens, this is a key quantitative measure in the design of a closed-loop controller to operate with the system concerned. This controller, operating through measurements of actual mean arterial pressure in comparison with demanded pressure, will stabilise the variable by adjustments of the infusion rate of the vasodilating agent. As is now well known, the method has proved entirely workable and successful in practice, and the next step – to provide for control of the second important determinant of LV function, myocardial contractility – is almost complete. The entire procedure thus points towards a range of similar new quantitative applications in therapeutic cardiology.

IN SUMMARY AND LOOKING AHEAD

Cardiological variables are often subject to substantial variability with a strong systematic component. Statistical procedures are vital. It is now known how to use statistics safely in this kind of situation; the method is quite general and it applies with particular force to quantitating pattern features of cardiological variables. Consequently, it makes good sense to think about statistical base-lines for all manner of cardiological variables and signals.

More base-line information is needed, some of which can only come from population studies. Ambulatory monitoring is one step in the necessary direction, needing its own special techniques of quantitation. The systematic preparation of guideline information on the properties of cardiological variables is another.

But when the patient must serve as his own control, we are into the quantitative complexities of trend detection and analysis, and ultimately automatic regulation. It is necessary to study the effects of variability in the evaluation of the patient system to be controlled, but, here again, the appropriate techniques have now been developed. Doubtless wider use of this approach will be made in the therapeutic application of automatic control in the future.

Other more speculative possibilities can be envisaged. It seems at least possible to use recent technological advances to convert passive implanted devices into more useful elements. For example, one imagines a heart valve prosthesis being provided with a transducer that would measure blood flow or blood pressure and that could be interrogated non-invasively. A second major early development will focus on automated image enhancement of ultrasonic and radiological images, using non-linear methods and perhaps drawing upon the perceptive skills of the radiologist (a rarely adopted but valuable component of the automated process); this certainly has the potential to improve vastly the utility of procedures for visualisation of cardiac structures. Third, a new generation of cardiological instruments can be anticipated that will include display of measurements at a resolution appropriate to the variable and include a statistical interface unit to estimate on a running basis, and use, where necessary, correlational structure and degrees of freedom information.

Finally, it seems possible that the use of dynamic ultrasonic or radiological information about ventricular wall movements and velocities in conjunction with LV pressure data, mathematical procedures, and anatomical information will permit estimates to be made of useful new indices – like the manner in which the myocardial oxygen supply–demand balance is distributed through the myocardium, and the pattern of intra-myocardial stress.

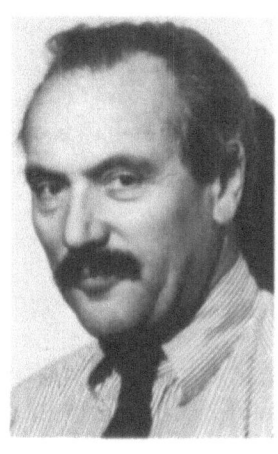

PAUL G. HUGENHOLTZ
W. A. H. ENGELSE / C. ZEELENBERG
M. R. HOARE / H. REIBER
SWAN PENG LIE / M. L. SIMOONS

Paul G. Hugenholtz is a professor of cardiology at the Medical Faculty in Rotterdam and professor of cardiology at the Inter-University Cardiologic Institute, Amsterdam. He serves on the editorial boards of seven journals. He is the secretary of the Board of the European Society of Cardiology, president of the Dutch Cardiac Society and member of the Board of the Dutch Heart Foundation.
His major research concerns the hemodynamic and electromotive behavior of the heart and the simplification of techniques for analysis of hemodynamic disorders. He has a special interest in computers in cardiology and in echocardiography.

Automation in cardiology

INTRODUCTION

The presentation during the Einthoven meeting fell into four parts: one dealing with the current status of automation in electrocardiographic processing; the second, the use of these techniques in intensive care; the third, the rapidly expanding field of image processing in medical imaging such as the automated contour recognition of coronary arteries and left ventricles; and finally a discussion of the improvement of interpretation of scintigrams obtained from gamma cameras. Since the available space in this publication is limited, it was elected to concentrate on two topics – the application of automation in intensive care, and the application of cardiac scintigrams – rather than to be superficial, and perhaps too brief, in covering all four.

To be complete, first here are a few words on each of the topics that are not included in the following text. The use of the digital computer in the processing of electrocardiograms is now common in several universities in the Netherlands. In Leiden, the Bonner program is used most frequently, in Rotterdam and Utrecht mostly the Pipberger VA 3.5, 3.7 program. In Rotterdam, the growth has been rapid from 17,074 electrocardiograms so processed in 1974 to 34,604 tracings in 1977. In the last two years, this growth has continued so that in 1980 more than 50,000 such ECGs will have been processed. Not all are taken from within the hospital; roughly 40% now come from several practices, occupational health services, and smaller hospitals in the immediate area. It is to be hoped that in the near future a common program will become available for all University hospitals.

99

The application of the smaller computer in image processing of X-ray pictures of the left ventricular outline and of the coronary arteries has been described elsewhere[1–6]. A brief overview follows here of our efforts to employ the computer in the nuclear field.

QUANTITATIVE ANALYSIS OF CARDIAC SCINTIGRAMS

Stress thallium-201 myocardial scintigraphy followed after 3–4 h by redistribution scintigraphy has been accepted as a clinically useful procedure for the detection of exercise-induced ischemia. An area with reduced thallium uptake after exercise may be due either to reversible ischemia or to a previous myocardial infarction. These two possibilities can be distinguished by comparison of the immediate postexercise image with the redistribution image[7]. In part of the patient population, it may not be clear from the visual interpretation of the analog or digital images whether redistribution has occurred or not; furthermore the extent of a defect is often difficult to determine.

To minimize the inter- and intraobserver variations in the interpretation of the scintigrams and to quantify the uptake defects, several computerized analysis methods have been published in the literature. Techniques have been developed for image registration of the exercise and rest thallium scintigrams, either under operator interaction enabling only translation[8], or from visually identifiable features ('landmarks') in the scintigrams enabling corrections for translation, rotation, scale, skew, as well as higher-order distortions[9]. Following another operator-interactive approach developed by Burow et al.[10], thallium defects are identified and scored by comparison of circumferential profiles of the nonregistered exercise and redistribution images with empirically determined normal limits.

We have developed a new technique for the computer processing of thallium-201 exercise/redistribution images with radioactive markers on the body to be used as landmarks[11–13]. In the development of this method, our goal has been to limit the role of the operator to 'controller' of the presented results with the possibility to interact in the quantification process, if the operator does not agree with the displayed results. This new technique is based on determining activity changes along a myocardial profile in the registered exercise and redistribution images. To facilitate circumferential profile analysis, the activity boundary of the exercise left ventricular structure is detected automatically. The procedure has been implemented on a DEC gamma-11 computer system. This technique has been shown to increase the sensitivity and specificity of interpretation of the scintigrams as compared with visual interpretation of the analog Polaroid images from the gamma camera or unprocessed images from the computer system[14].

100

DATA ACQUISITION AND ANALYSIS

In order to quantify the location and extent of thallium uptake defects, as well as the degree of redistribution, exercise and redistribution images need to be superimposed accurately. This can be achieved with the aid of two external markers (9.5 μCi cobalt-57 point sources) which are taped to the patient's chest. The positions are taken preferably at the left side of the heart, approximately 2 cm above and below the heart, respectively. These positions of the two point sources on the chest are marked by felt pen, so that exactly the same positions can be used for the redistribution images.

The scintigrams are acquired by using standard techniques. The patient performs a symptom-limited exercise test on a bicycle ergometer. One minute prior to maximal exercise 1.5–2.0 μCi Tl-201 is administered intravenously. Gated thallium scintigrams (10 frames in each cardiac cycle, 8-min acquisition period per view) are collected successively in the anterior, LAO-65, and LAO-45 orientations. Subsequently static thallium scintigrams are collected in the left lateral (LL) and LAO-25 views; these images contain 400,000 counts full field. After 3- to 4-h, redistribution imaging is performed in the same sequence. All studies are done with a Searle Pho Gamma V medium field gamma camera with a LEAP parallel-hole collimator. The three energy spectra of the camera are set as follows: channel 1: thallium 78 keV, 40% window; channel 2: cobalt 122 keV, 5% window; channel 3: thallium 167 keV, 20% window. Data are stored in the computer in 64×64 matrices.

After collection of all views from the exercise and redistribution studies, the data analysis program is initiated. Corresponding exercise and redistribution images are searched for in the patient file directory. For the gated studies, both the total images and the computed end-diastolic images are analyzed.

The analysis procedure is structured as a sequence of programs, which will be described in more detail in the following sections. First, the positions of the point sources in a pair of exercise and redistribution images are detected; from these x, y coordinates the redistribution image is translated and rotated such that it overlays the exercise image accurately. Next, the exercise image is filtered and a closed contour is detected along the activity distribution of the heart. From the exercise image and transformed redistribution image, a functional image is generated, which represents the percentage changes in activity between the exercise and redistribution images. Finally, quantification of the location and extent of perfusion defects is achieved by determining the activity changes in radial segments (6 degrees) from the geometric center of the closed contour along a myocardial profile in the bounded images. At a number of steps within the total analysis procedure, the user can interact with the software program if he is not satisfied with the intermediate results.

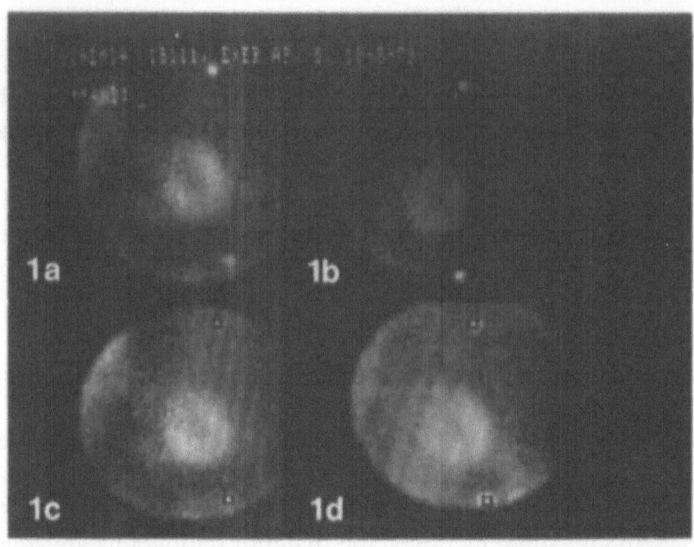

Fig. 1. (a and b) Corresponding exercise and redistribution images. (c) The exercise image with the point sources eliminated and marked. (d) The transformed redistribution image.

IMAGE SUPERIMPOSITION

To quantify differences in uptake patterns in corresponding exercise and redistribution images collected at different times, the two images must be registered accurately. For our clinical thallium studies, we use a parallel-hole collimator featuring constant magnification as a function of the collimator-to-object distances. This implies that changes in scale do not occur. The gamma camera produces a two-dimensional projection of a three-dimensional object (the heart). Rotation of the heart in a plane parallel to the plane of the collimeter thus can be corrected for with external markers. However, rotations of the heart in planes not parallel to the plane of the collimator will produce distortions that are difficult to correct for. We believe that with accurate repositioning of the patient, the camera head and the point sources for the redistribution images, the latter rotational errors are of minor importance, taking into account the relatively low resolution of the scintigrams.

From these observations, we have decided to correct the images only for rotation and translation in the plane parallel to the plane of the collimator, thus requiring two radioactive markers.

The locations of the point sources in the computer-stored scintigrams are detected automatically; the detection algorithm is based on the known point source response. Details of this algorithm and of the transformation procedure have been described elsewhere [13].

Figure 1 presents the results of this transformation. The original thallium

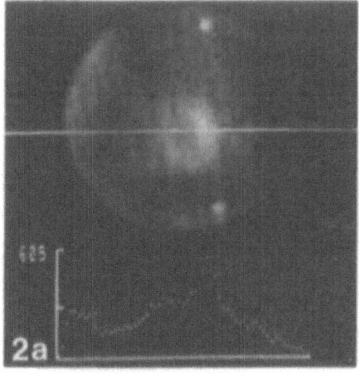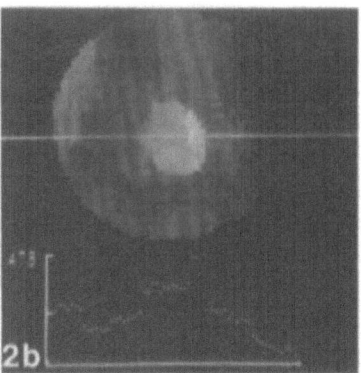

Fig. 2. (a) The activity plot along a line across the myocardium before the filter is applied. (b) The result of the nonlinear filter.

exercise and redistribution images with the cobalt point sources are shown in Figure 1a and b, respectively. In the exercise image of Figure 1c, the point sources have been detected, eliminated, and the positions marked with single bright points for optimal display purposes. Similarly, Figure 1d gives the redistribution image after it has been transformed to match the exercise image.

CONTOUR DETECTION

In clinical practice, the number of counts collected in thallium images is relatively low, which results in large statistical variations. To decrease these statistical noise influences to an acceptable level before a contour detection algorithm is applied, a nonlinear spatial filter is used. This filter smooths the noise in the object and the background, while it enhances the edges. Figure 2 shows the result of the nonlinear filter applied on the exercise image of Figure 1. Delineation of the heart contour has improved significantly.

To detect the activity boundary of the heart, a contour-tracking algorithm has been developed based on search techniques with backup [13]. The contour detection problem is defined as a minimalization problem of an evaluation function applying a first-derivative function. In Figure 3, the results of this contour detection algorithm on the filtered image are shown.

FUNCTIONAL IMAGES AND SEGMENTATION

After the images have been registered and the heart contour found, the changes in thallium distribution from the exercise to the redistribution images can be visualized and described quantitatively. The heart contour detected in the exercise image is superimposed in the redistribution image. If the heart contour does not seem to fit the redistribution activity structure correctly, the operator can interactively shift the redistribution image with respect to the

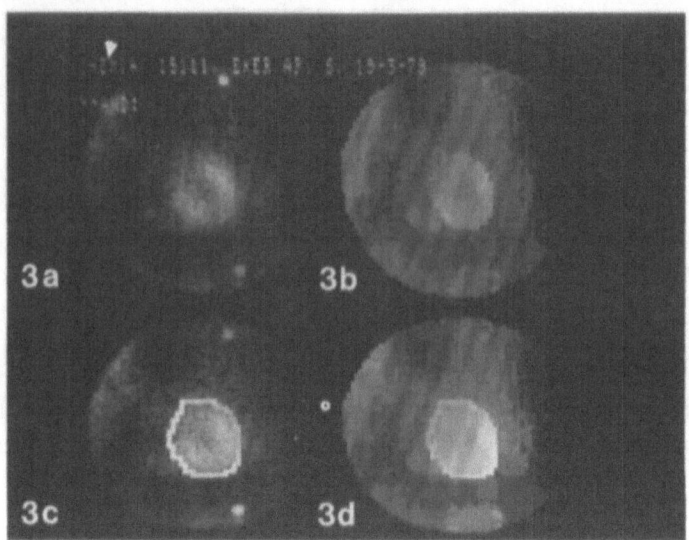

Fig. 3. (a and b) The original and filtered image, respectively. (c and d) The detected contour is superimposed in the images of a and b, respectively.

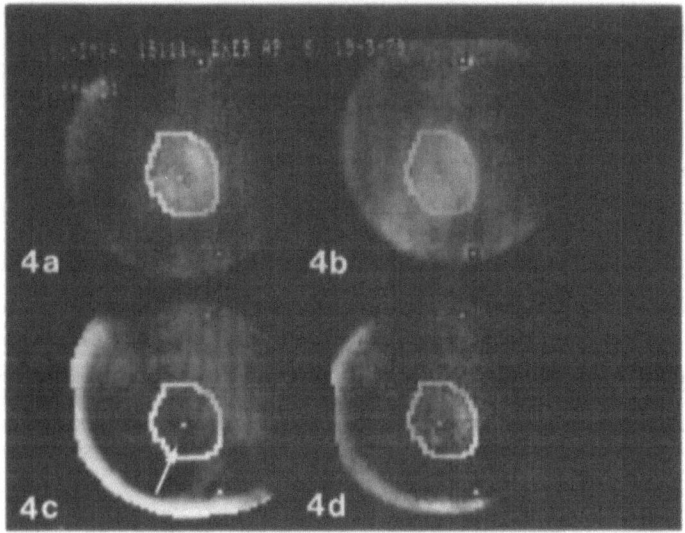

Fig. 4. (a) The exercise image. (b) The corresponding transformed redistribution image. (c) The functional image. (d) The subtraction image. The arrow indicates an area in which redistribution has occurred.

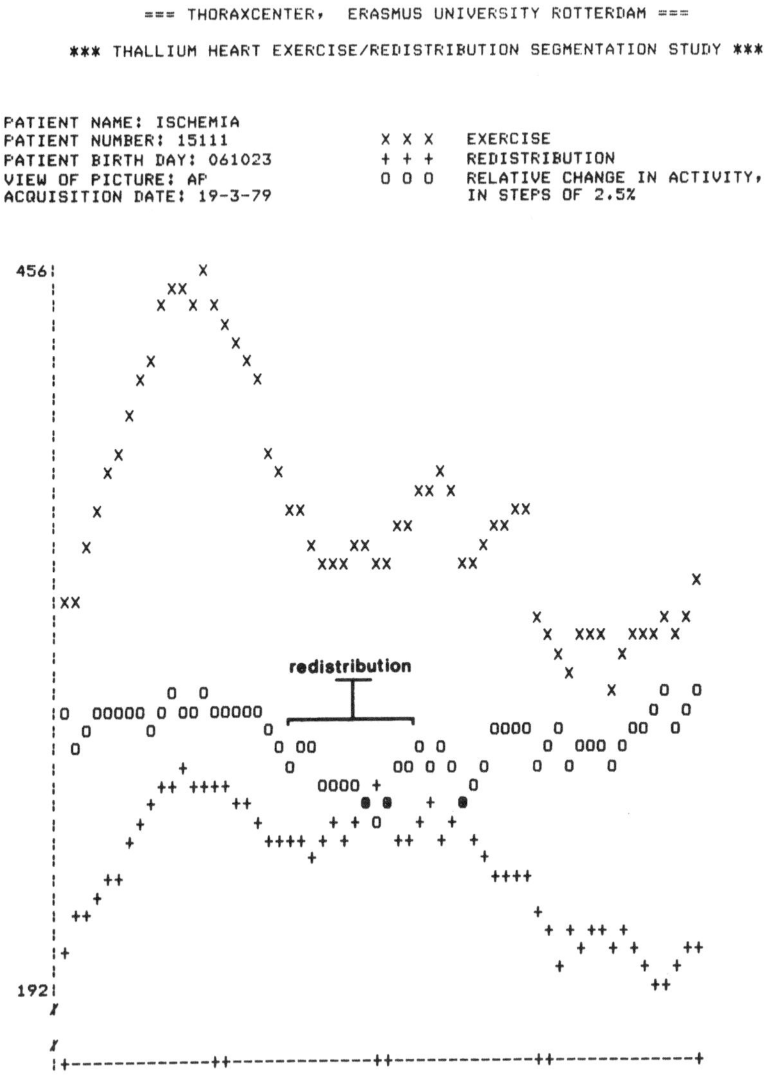

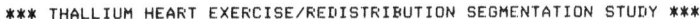

=== THORAXCENTER, ERASMUS UNIVERSITY ROTTERDAM ===

*** THALLIUM HEART EXERCISE/REDISTRIBUTION SEGMENTATION STUDY ***

```
PATIENT NAME: ISCHEMIA
PATIENT NUMBER: 15111          X X X   EXERCISE
PATIENT BIRTH DAY: 061023      + + +   REDISTRIBUTION
VIEW OF PICTURE: AP            O O O   RELATIVE CHANGE IN ACTIVITY,
ACQUISITION DATE: 19-3-79              IN STEPS OF 2.5%


   456:                    X
      !              XX
      !            X  X  X
      !                   X
      !                    X
      !          X        X
      !        X           X
      !
      !      X
      !
      !     X        X
      !    X        X             X
      !                          XX X
      !   X         XX                    XX
      !                  XX        XX
      ! X          X  XX         X
      !            XXX  XX      XX
      !                                              X
      !XX
      !                               X        X X
      !                             X XXX  XXX X
      !                             X     X
      !                             X
      !            O  O    redistribution    X   O  O
      !                          ┬                 O O
      !O  00000 O 00 00000 ┌─────┴─────┐      0000  0   00 O
      ! O     O          O              0 00    0     00 O
      ! O                    O 00          O O     O 000 O
      !        +                O       00 O O  O   O  O   O
      !     ++ ++++           0000 +          O
      !      +       ++        ● ●      + ●
      !       +          +    + + O     + +
      !       +        ++++ + +    ++  +  +
      !                     +                +
      !    ++                              ++++
      !     +
      !   ++                           +
      !  +                           + + ++ +
      ! +                              + + +     ++
      ! +                            +      +  +
   192:                                    ++
     ⌡
     ⌡
     !+-------------++-------------++-------------++-------------+
```

Fig. 5. Plot of the average segment activity of the images in Figure 4a–c.

stationary contour in horizontal and vertical directions. Such a misfit is usually due to inaccurate repositioning of the point sources during the redistribution collection. If the acquisition periods for the two images are different, the images are normalized for scan time. From the exercise and redistribution images, two new images are generated. A subtraction image is defined as (exercise image) − (redistribution image) and a functional image as [(subtraction image)/(exercise image)] × 100%. The latter image represents the changes in activity between the exercise and redistribution images as a percentage of the exercise image. The resulting four images are shown in Figure 4. The relatively dark areas within the heart boundary in the functional image are areas where redistribution has occurred.

Quantification of the location and extent of uptake defects is achieved by determining the average activity within radial segments in the exercise and redistribution images. These radial segments are defined with respect to the geometric center of the closed contour; each segment subtends 6 degrees. The segmentation starts at 12 o'clock moving counterclockwise. In the final output, the average activity in each segment for the exercise and redistribution images is plotted as a function of the segment number (Fig. 5). A third function is calculated and plotted, which represents the relative activity change in a segment. The marked dip in this curve in Figure 5 corresponds with the dark area in Figure 4 representing an area where redistribution has occurred.

INITIAL CLINICAL RESULTS

To determine the sensitivity of the described method, the scintigrams of a group of 25 patients with significant coronary artery disease were interpreted by two cardiologists in the following sequence:

a) On bases of the analog Polaroid pictures from the gamma camera, corresponding exercise and redistribution images for the five views were visually judged as normal or abnormal. A patient was defined as abnormal if a perfusion defect could be distinguished. From the total group of 25 patients, 11 patients were found to be abnormal and 14 normal.
b) For the three gated views, the end-diastolic images were reconstructed by the computer. Visual inspection of these images resulted in diagnosing the same group of 11 abnormal patients to be abnormal while three other patients were also classified as abnormal.
c) Functional images and segmentation profiles were generated from the three gated views, both total images and end-diastolic images. In an additional five patients from the remaining group of 11 'normal' patients, perfusion defects could be found from these data. All 14 'abnormal' patients, classified before, were again found to be abnormal.

Therefore, the final results from the different ways of interpreting the thallium images in this group of 25 patients indicate that 19 were classified as abnormal and six patients as normal. No further information was gained from the functional images and segmentation profiles of the end-diastolic images compared with the total images.

106

From the above results the preliminary remark can be made that the sensitivity of exercise and redistribution thallium imaging increases with the degree of quantification of these images. In addition to this application, in the near future we will see improvements in processing of echocardiograms, halter cardiograms, and exercise electrocardiograms, and here the most rapid growth in application of microcomputers can be expected in the next few years. Now, let us turn our attention to the main body of the presentation.

THE UNIBED MONITORING SYSTEM

The last decade has seen some significant advances in the management and care of the critically ill patient. One major advance was the introduction of highly specialized units dedicated to the care of such specific conditions as coronary incident or shock. While the medical problems encountered in these units vary widely, the managerial and technical aspects exhibit many com-

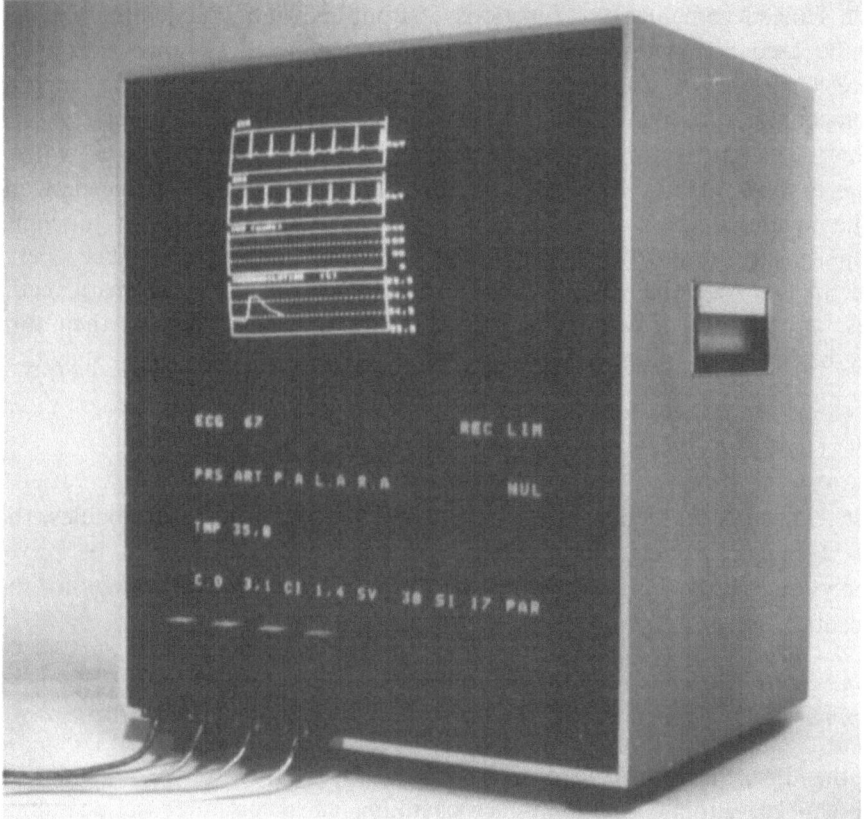

Fig. 6. The Unibed.

mon elements. The patients require constant surveillance from the clinical staff; for optimal therapy they also need frequent, accurately detailed measurement of many physiological parameters and signals. This means that modern technology in general, and computers in particular, have come to play an increasingly important role and today from an integral, not to say intrinsic, part of the concept of 'intensive care.'

The Thoraxcenter in Rotterdam has been working with computer-aided patient monitoring since the end of the 1960s. Two in-house systems were developed, a 'large' system for general ICU monitoring[15] and a 'small' system for ECG monitoring only, for pre-coronary care[16]. Experience with these systems had involved many of the problems previously described, and had led to considerable dissatisfaction with the centralized approach. The system now operational at the Thoraxcenter incorporates many points intended to reduce or eliminate the difficulties encountered with the previous generation. The system was designed as a hierarchical network of microcomputers[17]. The base level is made up of a single type of unit, the Unibed[18]. Each Unibed combines the functions of front-end and signal processor and can be used completely stand-alone (Fig. 6). In practice, however, one or more Unibeds are usually coupled via a standard serial link to another microcomputer at the nurse station to provide time-trend graphics, strip recording, alarm setting, and other centralized functions. Should a Unibed cease to work, it may be replaced without affecting the rest of the network while failure of the nurse station will cut out the nurse-station functions (graphics, strip recorder, etc.) without endangering the bedside Unibed operation. In this way, the system attempts to provide one of the primary requisites for this type of equipment, 'fail-soft.' The nurse stations in their turn may be linked to a higher level, say for data bases and long-term statistics.

THE UNIBED

Each Unibed is made up of four basic elements: the command modules, the LSI-11 microcomputer, the video display, and the Unibox with its power supply, mounting rack for LSI-11, and command modules and sockets for the transducer plugs.

Command module and transducer plugs

To the user, the command module appears as the intelligent component of the Unibed, although it is in fact operating as a computer peripheral. A Unibox can contain a number of identical and completely interchangeable command modules (typically four or six). A command module has two

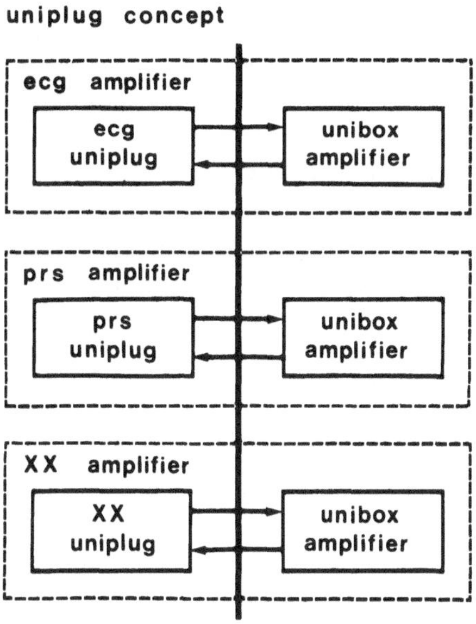

uniplug concept

Fig. 7. The Uniplug concept.

identifiable tasks: the patient interface and the user interface. The patient interface consists of a very versatile four-channel amplifier, analog multiplex, or analog-to-digital converter, a 16-bit digital interface, and all the required patient isolation circuitry. Because of its unique structure, the analog subsystem is capable of handling signals from many different physiological transducers. The signal-dependent characteristics such as gain, input impedance, and frequency response are determined by circuitry in the actual signal plug. Figure 7 illustrates this structure whereby, for example, when an ECG plug is plugged into any command module, they together provide a complete ECG amplifier. Plugs are designed for handling signals from a single-lead ECG (with defibrillation protection and electrode loose detection), a pressure transducer, a dual temperature probe, and a thermodilution cardiac output catheter. The signal plug also generates an identification code on four of the digital input lines. Whenever the executive detects a coded plug, it activates the corresponding firmware application module.

User interface

The most striking feature of the command module, and of the Unibox as a whole, is that there are no buttons, or meters of any kind, but only sockets for the transducer plugs. With the exception of signal traces, which appear on the video display unit, all communication and interaction with the Unibed

109

makes use of the touch-sensitive LED character display ('touch-line'). Since the latter can act as a computer terminal, it is available to the application programs for the presentation of numeric data, text information, alarm messages, action requests, etc. Continuously updated values of the more important parameters are displayed here whenever a signal is montored. Interaction between system and user is basically initiated and controlled by the computer. Once an application has been activated by plugging in the required signal, the user is guided through procedures by prompts from the application program appearing on the touch-line. Certain actions, such as limit setting can be performed at any time and are initiated whenever the computer senses that a character of a given command module has been touched.

Video display unit

The video display unit is, like the command module, a computer peripheral. It operates entirely under control of the microcomputer. The unit is capable of displaying four signal traces with calibration lines, as well as 32 lines of 32 characters each of textual information. Signal traces are displayed with normalized gain, mnemonic identification, and an indication of the exact range.

The microcomputer

The microcomputer is responsible for controlling the entire system, handling the signal display, and providing the link to the nurse station, if required. The system uses a Digital Equipment LSI-11 microcomputer, chosen for its flexible architecture, range of support software, and the availability of a large number of compatible PDP-11 computer systems already in use at the development site. Both monitor and application programs are 'firmware' programmable read-only memory (EPROM) with random-access memory (RAM) as working area. New applications are debugged by using a development system with MOS read/write memory and down-line loading from a 'host' PDP-11/10. Once debugged, adding a new application is a matter of programming the EPROM, plugging it into the LSI-11, and adding a suitably coded transducer plug with appropriate signal conditioning.

Firmware

The Unibed firmware consists of a system executive and a set of application programs for handling the various physiological monitoring functions. Some

110

applications (ECG, pressures, temperatures, fluid output) are primarily intended for continuous monitoring while others are by nature relatively infrequent measurements (thermodilution cardiac output). Some 'continuous' measurements may be performed only intermittently (certain pressures), depending on the protocol to be followed by the nurse. The following example of an application (cardiac output measured by thermodilution) gives a good impression of the way in which the system interacts with the user. The module is activated whenever the executive detects the connection of a properly coded plug. The command module responds by displaying the cardiac output signal designator and a key for changing preset measurement parameters.

✳ ✳ ✳

C.O   PAR

Touching the designator 'key' starts the measurement and the command module then directs the procedure.

C.O   INJECT   10 mL AT   0 t   PAR

When the application program detects an acceptable thermodilution curve, it will integrate the signal and compute the cardiac output using the Stewart-Hamilton formula.

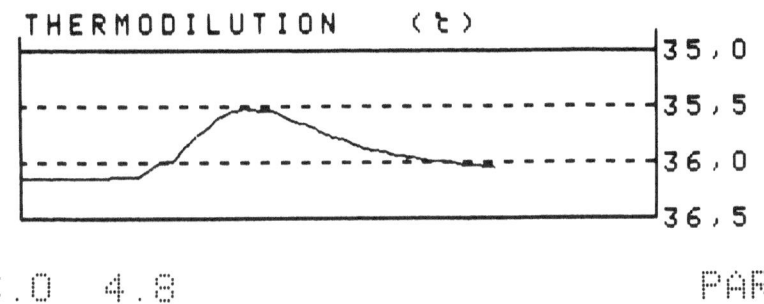

C.O   4.8   PAR

Communication between application modules is possible. The thermodilution module checks the ECG module to see if the heart rate is available and, if so, calculates the stroke volume.

ECG   74   LIM

C.O   4.8 SV 65   PAR

The values for the patient's body-surface area, the temperature and volume of the injectate, and the catheter number can be modified by touching the PAR key. The module will respond by displaying the default numbers; touching the individual digits will increment their values.

```
C.O BS 0.0 0   TI 0 0   VI 1 0   7F

C.O BS 1.0 0   TI 0 0   VI 1 0   7F

C.O BS 2.0 0   TI 0 0   VI 1 0   7F
```

Returning to the cardiac output display, by touching the C.O. key, will recalculate the values by using the newly entered numbers. Now, using the body-surface area, the application module also computes the cardiac and stroke index.

```
C.O   4.8 CI   2.4 SV 65 SI 32 PAR
```

CONCLUSION

Over the last two decades, computers have become an integral part of the concept 'intensive care', and few large CCUs or ICUs lack some type of computer assistance. Third-generation, microcomputer-based systems are helping to solve many of the earlier problems. Features such as touch-sensitive keys or screens (eliminating keyboards) and integrated front-end with automatic gain control, together with simplified procedures, are greatly increasing user acceptance. The basic signals monitored are virtually unchanged. The pattern-recognition programs for monitoring which are in general use today are still susceptible to artifact. Yet ECG quality, for instance, is still mainly a question of correct electrode placement, ensuring good contact and keeping the patient quiet. Pressures and cardiac output are monitored with in-dwelling catheters, with all their attendant risks. The techniques available for improving signal quality may be unpleasant for the patient and may not be completely without risk. Noninvasive methods for pressure and flow measurement are still in their infancy and the problems of new electrode systems, such as esophageal leads, are far from solved. Yet now that sufficient computer power can be available at every bed, it is surely time to start concentrating on new techniques and new applications as well as on improving existing ones. Computer systems should be used to improve patient care in

112

the wider sense of these words. We must await in-depth evaluations of third-generation systems to see whether or not they fulfill this aim and provide a truly valuable aid for the clinical staff of the CCU.

SUMMARY

In the oral presentation, a number of projects were described in which automation has played a major role at the Thoraxcenter in Rotterdam. Two of these are described in this paper: the Unibed monitoring system and the quantitative analysis of cardiac scintigrams. In the latter, a method has been presented for the automated border recognition in thallium images and the subsequent quantitative assessment of uptake defects from exercise and rest (redistribution) thallium images. Preliminary results show that the sensitivity to detect differences in uptake patterns between exercise and redistribution thallium scintigrams by this method is higher than by visual interpretation of the images. The specificity of this method remains to be determined, as well as its relative superiority over exercise ECG analysis.

The Unibed patient-monitoring system represents a new approach to the design of medical instrumentation based upon recent advances in microcomputer and related large-scale integration technology. This system is intended to replace an entire range of traditional monitoring devices with a single general-purpose unit capable of recognizing the nature of the signal source and performing appropriately. All of the usual switches, knobs, dials, and meters have been replaced by a touch-sensitive character display. The hardware responsible for physiological signal analysis, information display, and user interaction is actually a set of firmware which gives the system its functional personality and transforms it from a compact process-control system into a useful medical instrument. Twenty systems have been installed at the intensive care units of the Thoraxcenter of the Dijkzigt University Hospital, Rotterdam, the Netherlands.

REFERENCES

1. Slager CJ, Reiber JHC, Schuurbiers JCH, Meester GT (1978) Contouromat – A hard-wired left ventricular angio-processing system. I. Design and application. Comput Biomed Res 11:491–502.
2. Reiber JHC, Slager CJ, Schuurbiers JCH, Meester GT (1978) Contouromat – A hard-wired left ventricular angio-processing system. II. Performance evaluation. Comput Biomed Res 11:503–523.
3. Reiber JHC, Booman F, Tan HS, Slager CJ, Schuurbiers JCH, Gerbrands JJ, Meester GT (1978) A cardiac image analysis system. Objective quantitative processing of angiocardiograms. Proc Comput Cardiol, pp 239–242.

4. Reiber JHC, Booman F, Tan HS, Lie SP, Gerbrands JJ, Slager CJ, Schuurbiers JCH, Meester GT, Simoons ML (1979) Kwantitatieve beeldverwerking in de cardiologie. Proceedings Post-academische Cursus, Beeldverwerking en Patroonherkenning, Delft, 16-18 May, pp 216-243.

5. Reiber JHC, Booman F, Tan HS, Gerbrands JJ, Slager CJ, Schuurbiers JCH, Meester GT (1979) Computer processing of coronary occlusions from X-ray arteriograms. In: Proceedings 6th International Conference on Information Processing in Medical Imaging, Paris (in press)

6. Booman F, Reiber JHC, Gerbrands JJ, Slager CJ, Schuurbiers JCH, Meester GT (1979) Quantitative analysis of coronary occlusions from coronary cine-angiograms. Proc Comput Cardiol (in press)

7. Pohost GM, Zir LM, Moore RH, McKusick KA, Guiney TE, Beller GA (1977) Differentiation of transiently ischemic from infarcted myocardium by serial imaging after a single dose of thallium-201. Circulation 55:294-302

8. Williams DL, Ritchie JL, Hamilton GW (1978) Implementation of a digital image superposition algorithm for radionuclide images: An assessment of its accuracy and reproducibility. J Nucl Med 19:316-319

9. Singh M, Frei W, Shibata T, et al. (1977) A digital technique for accurate change detection in nuclear medical images with application to myocardial perfusion studies using thallium-201. IEEE Trans Nucl Sci NS-26:565-575

10. Burow RD, Pond M, Schafer AW, Becker L (1979) Circumferetial profiles: a new method for computer analysis of thallium-201 myocardial perfusion images. J Nucl Med 20:771-777

11. Lie SP (1979) Kwantitatieve analyse van thallium scintigrammen [in Dutch]. Thesis, Delft University of Technology, Delft

12. Reiber JHC, Lie SP, Simoons ML, et al. (1979) Quantitative analysis of thallium-201 myocardial images. Proc Eur Soc Cardiol Workshop: Use of isotopes [Abstr]. Tours, 21-22 May, p 66

13. Lie SP, Reiber JHC, Simoons ML, Withagen AJA, Gerbrands JJ (1979) Quantification of the location and extent of defects in thallium-201 uptake and redistribution patterns. Proc Comp Cardiol (in press)

14. Simmons ML (1979) Kwantitatieve analyse van het thalliumscintigram. Symposium Nucleaire Diagnostiek, Utrecht, 19-20 October

15. Zeelenberg C, Hoare MR, Engelse WAH, Hagemeijer F, Hugenholtz PG (1974) Arrhythmia monitoring at the Thoraxcentrum, Rotterdam. Proc Comput Cardiol, IEEE Comput Soc, pp 203-204

16. Zeelenberg C, Deutsch LS, Engelse WAH, Corbeij HMA (1976) Experiences with implementing ARGUS in a cardiac surveillance unit. Proc Trends Comput Processed ECG's. Amsterdam, p 31

17. Zeelenberg C, Engelse WAH, Deutsch LS (1977) A hierarchical patient monitoring computer network. Proc Cardiol, IEEE Comput Soc, pp 439-444

18. Deutsch LS, Engelse WAH, Zeelenberg C, van der Voorde F, Hugenholtz PG (1977) The Unibed patient monitoring system: a new approach for a new technology. Med Instrum (Baltimore) 11:274-277

J. B. VAN DER SCHOOT

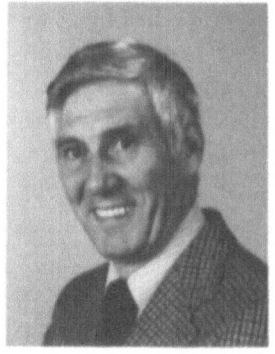

Jan B. van der Schoot is professor of nuclear medicine at the University of Amsterdam and is head of the Department of Nuclear Medicine at the University Hospital, Wilhelmina Gasthuis. His initial training was in internal medicine, but he has been working in the field of nuclear medicine since 1959. During the past few years, his main interests have been nuclear cardiology and labeled blood cells. The work in nuclear cardiology has always been done in close cooperation with the Department of Cardiology and has led to a number of publications on the use of thallium-201 in coronary heart disease.

Nuclear cardiology

Noninvasive techniques for diagnosis of cardiac disease have long been known, and electrocardiography, cardiac fluoroscopy and, later, phonocardiography were added in the first half of this century. With cardiac catheterization and angiocardiography a period of invasive techniques started. Echocardiography enlarged the possibilities of noninvasive cardiac diagnosis and its development in the last ten years has been very successful. With the use of radioactive tracers, another methodology of noninvasive cardiac diagnosis has been introduced into clinical practice and, due to the quantitative nature of radionuclide counting, it is especially apt to give numerical values for blood flow, cardiac function, and myocardial metabolism. Gated blood pool techniques enable us to study wall motion, ejection fraction, and ejection and filling rates. Myocardial scintigraphy enables us to diagnose myocardial infarction in cases of doubtful history and inconclusive ECG.

As early as 1927, Blumgart used a radioactive tracer, bismuth-214 (a radioactive daughter of radium), to measure the circulation time between arm and heart. The second conclusion in his article states: 'because of the simplicity of the procedure... the method is well suited to the determination of this test in man,' an aphorism which still holds true today for cardiovascular nuclear medicine.

In 1948, Prinzmetal described radiocardiography using a GM counter and radioactive sodium. The normal curve shows separately the passage of a radioactive bolus through the right and left heart. A prolongation of the passage through the left ventricle may indicate a dilatation of that ventricle.

Of great importance to the development of nuclear cardiology has been the introduction of new radiopharmaceuticals, enabling the use of larger quantities of radioactivity without much increase in the radiation dose to the patient, and enabling us to visualize blood pool and myocardium. Another important stimulus for the development of nuclear cardiology has been the sophistication of the detection instruments and the on-line use of minicomputer systems. With such a gamma camera–computer system, one can study the passage of a radioactive bolus through heart and lungs, and register all the information. From the computer memory, one can afterward reconstruct in successive frames of different duration the passage of the radioactive bolus and view the passage in cine mode or in separate scintiscans. Choosing a region of interest over the left ventricle, one can follow the activity in the left ventricle. With a framing rate of 2 frames per second, one sees the passage of the bolus through the left ventricle as on the radiocardiogram with the technique of Prinzmetal. With a framing rate of 50 frames per second, one can

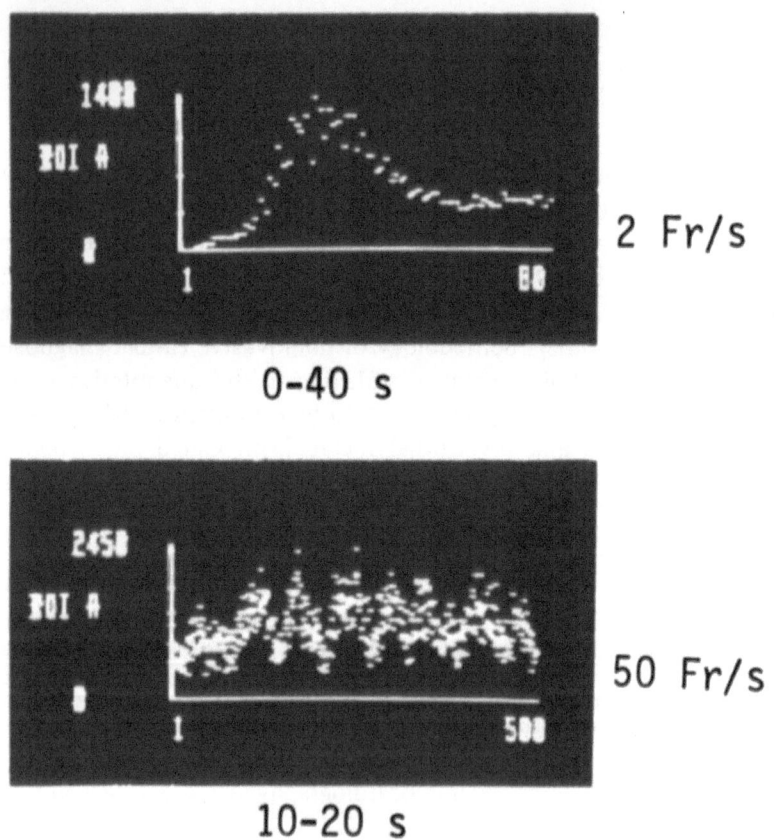

Fig. 1. Top: Passage of bolus through left ventricle. Framing rate 2/s. Bottom: Visualization of ventricular contractions using a rapid framing rate (50/s).

see changes of activity proportional to changes of ventricular volume, due to successive ventricular contractions (Fig. 1).

Another technique is gated blood pool scintigraphy. After intravenous injection of a radioactive blood pool tracer, we wait until the tracer has been evenly distributed in the blood and then computer-assisted scans of the heart are made. Triggering on the R wave of the ECG, we sample successive fractions from each of 100–1000 heart cycles, adding together in the computer the corresponding fractions of the different cycles. In such a way in the computer a representative cycle is constructed, consisting mostly of 20–50 fractions or frames. In this representative cycle, we can study wall motion, for instance, by viewing the consecutive frames in cine mode, and we can calculate ejection fraction after quantitation of the activity in the left ventricle.

We can also study the first pass of a radioactive tracer through heart and lungs for the presence of an abnormal shunt. A right-to-left shunt may be detected by early filling of the left ventricle. A left-to-right shunt can be detected by the early recirculation of the activity in the right ventricle and lungs. Such an early recirculation of the activity in the lungs can be studied by a time-activity curve of the periphery of the lungs. In the case of a left-to-right shunt, one sees a hump on the downslope, indicating early recirculation. Using a computer program, one can extrapolate and subtract the first circulation from the time activity curve actually found and quantitate the recirculation. In this way one can detect shunts as low as 10%.

Using invasive techniques of coronary catheterization and injection of radioactive gases (^{133}Xe, ^{81m}Kr) or microspheres, myocardial blood flow can be directly studied and even quantitated. However, regional myocardial perfusion can also be studied after a simple intravenous injection of an appropriate radiotracer. Different cations, such as ^{43}K, ^{129}Cs, ^{81}Rb, ^{201}Tl, ^{13}NH$_4^+$, are extracted from the coronary blood flow with extraction efficiencies of up to 85% and, according to the Sapirstein principle, the primary distribution of these tracer substances in different organs and different parts of the myocardium depends on the regional blood flow. Fatty acids labeled with ^{123}I or ^{11}C are also concentrated in the myocardium by metabolic concentration. Using ^{11}C, one can study tomographic scintiscans of the heart by using a positron emission tomograph. Studies with tomographic accessories to gamma cameras and using gamma-emitting isotopes are now approaching clinical practice. Other radiotracers are concentrated in the infarcted myocardium. Figure 2 gives a ^{201}Tl scan and a ^{99m}Tc-pyrophosphate scan of the same patient. Thallium-201 is taken in the normal myocardium with an anteroseptal defect due to an anteroseptal myocardial infarction, whereas the pyrophosphate scan shows accumulation of activity in the infarcted myocardium. With ^{201}Tl, the right ventricle is mostly not visualized.

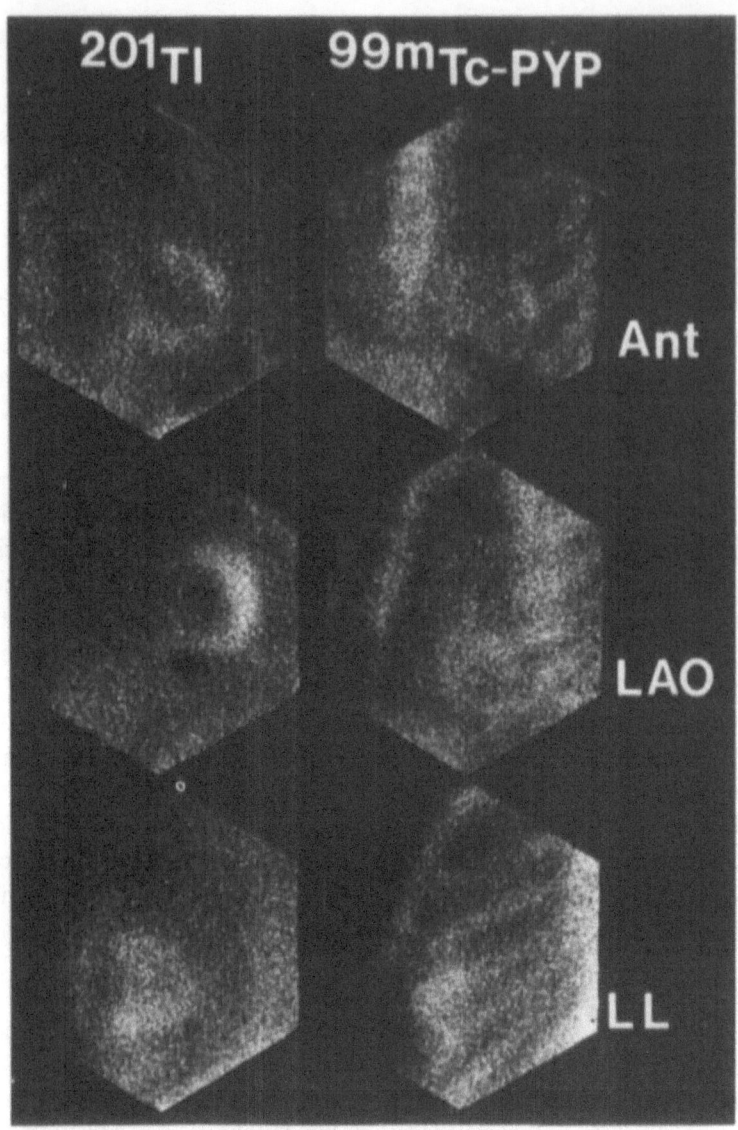

Fig. 2. Left: Thallium-201 scintigraphy showing an anteroseptal defect. Right: Technetium-99m pyrophosphate scan of the same patient showing accumulation of activity in the anteroseptal region.

In a series of 78 consecutive patients with an acute inferior infarction of the left ventricle, all had a defect on the thallium scan but only 64 had a positive pyrophosphate scan. All these patients were scanned in the first 24 h after onset of symptoms with thallium-201, and the pyrophosphate scans were performed at least 24 h after onset of symptoms with a mean time at 32 h. In 24–64 patients with a positive pyrophosphate scan, an accumulation of the

118

pyrophosphate complex in the right ventricle was also found, indicating an extension of the infarction in the right ventricle in 37% of these 64 patients. Only one of these 24 patients with pyrophosphate accumulation in the right ventricle showed a right-sided heart failure. This latter patient showed a greater uptake of the pyrophosphate in the right ventricle than the other patients in this series. Right ventricular involvement in acute inferior wall infarctions seems to be relatively frequent but is not necessarily associated with severe right heart failure. A difference in sensitivity for the detection of acute myocardial infarction by thallium and pyrophosphate scintigraphy was found in this series. For pyrophosphate scintigraphy, relatively early scanning after onset of symptoms may have influenced the relatively low percentage of positive pyrophosphate scans found. The pyrophosphate scan mostly becomes positive 12–24 h after onset of infarction. However, it may take 4–5 days before one obtains a positive pyrophosphate scan, probably due to a delayed collateral flow reaching the area of the irreversibly damaged myocardium, a delay due to extensive coronary artery disease.

We have found ^{201}Tl scintigraphy very sensitive for the detection of acute myocardial infarction, especially in the first day after onset of symptoms, that is, in the period when serum enzyme determinations are not yet available. In the first 6 h after onset of an infarction, we hardly miss any AMI, but between 6 and 24 h, we can miss a small, especially nontransmural, infarction. We can also localize the infarction with thallium-201. According to the localization of the defect, anteroseptal, anterolateral, inferior, or inferoposterior, different myocardial infarctions can be recognized. We can also localize the infarction in cases of altered intraventricular conduction, hampering or making impossible the electrocardiographic diagnosis of acute myocardial infarction. A defect on the thallium scan does not necessarily imply an acute myocardial infarction, but can also be due to scar tissue of an old myocardial infarction, cardiomyopathy, or transient myocardial ischemia.

The high sensitivity of thaillium-201 scintigraphy in fresh AMI is certainly partly due to concomitant ischemia in the acute phase, as can be seen in repeated studies after days 1 and 8. The disappearance or diminution of a clear defect in this time period indicates the recovery of an ischemic zone accompanying the acute infarction. We are now studyng the effect of vasodilating drugs for the diagnosis of imminent infarction; 15 min after sublingual nitroglycerin a defect on the thallium scan can disappear, indicating an improved perfusion in that area.

Another important indication for the use of thallium-201 is exercise scintigraphy. Thallium-201 is injected during maximal exercise, and scanning is started immediately. At first we used two thallium-201 injections: one for the exercise study and one after an interval of a few days for the rest study. Now we are using only one injection and studying the redistribution of thallium-201 after 2 h. Defects found directly after exercise may be absent on the scans made in rest. These defects were then due to transient exercise-induced ischemia on the basis of chronic coronary disease. Using the latter thallium-201 redistribution technique in 101 patients referred for coronary angiography, we found a sensitivity of 88% and a specificity of 93% for the detection of coronary artery disease. Compared with stress electrocardiography (sensitivity 83%, specificity 68%), the results of thallium-201 stress scintigraphy were apparently better, especially the specificity, which means fewer false positive results.

On the basis of our earlier experience with thallium-201 in acute myocardial infarction, we have used thallium-201 scintigraphy in our admittance policy for the coronary care unit, especially in patients with atypical history and inconclusive ECG. In our first group of 203 such patients, 87 were allowed to go home on the basis of a negative thallium-201 scintiscan. Only one of these patients had a small intramural infarction according to enzyme determinations, which were made on all patients the next day. When the pre-coronary care unit (PCU) was installed in Amsterdam in the Department of Cardiology for the selection of patients to be admitted to the coronary care unit (CCU), a cardiovascular nuclear medicine facility was incorporated into the PCU. In the first year, only 21% of about 3000 patients were admitted from the PCU to the CCU, and 71.4% of these patients admitted had an acute myocardial infarction. Since thallium-201 scintigraphy with and without nitroglycerin played an important role in equivocal cases, the high percentage AMI in the group of patients admitted to the CCU was due in part to the presence of the nuclear medicine facility in the PCU.

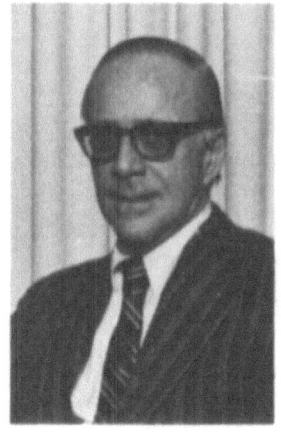

HERBERT L. ABRAMS

Herbert L. Abrams, born in 1920, was professor of radiology at the Stanford University School of Medicine till 1967 and thereafter held the same post at Harvard Medical School, where he is the chief radiologist at Peter Bent Brigham Hospital in Boston. His main interest over the years has been angiography of heart and vessels, both experimentally and clinically. He is the editor of the standard textbook of angiography and has contributed to numerous innovations in cineangiography, selective catheterization, renovascular hypertension, and computed tomography.

Angiocardiography

Angiocardiography, by definition, is the Roentgen contrast examination of the cardiovascular system. As a practical and widely applied method, it has moved by leaps and bounds from the early period in the late thirties of intravenous injection with single films, to cineangiocardiography and selective angiocardiography with multiple films in the forties and fifties, to biplane examinations with rapid cassette changers in the early fifties, and finally to biplane image amplified cineangiocardiography in the late fifties.

On a more personal note, I first become involved in angiocardiography in 1947, while training in radiology at Stanford University. By 1954, we had performed hundreds of angiocardiograms and, in the following year, Kaplan and I published our monograph on *Angiocardiographic Interpretation in Congenital Heart Disease* [1]. With the introduction of open-heart surgery at Stanford in 1955, we developed a strong focus on the assessment of operable heart disease [2–6], an interest which has continued through the years. Our first image-amplified biplane cineangiocardiograms were done in 1957 [7], and we have had the pleasure of observing and participating in the technical and scholarly developments in diagnostic cardiovascular radiology for three decades. What an exciting time it has been! How much safer and more precise have our diagnostic tools become!

Within the framework of this brief view of the present and future of the method, I will deal with the range of advances of the modern era in summary fashion, with the exception of those which are most recent, most provocative, and most likely to move on to further developments. Using the definition literally, the potential of contrast-enhanced cardiac computed tomography will also be assessed.

121

TECHNICAL DEVELOPMENTS

As angiocardiography became more widely applied in the sixties and late seventies, and particularly with the impetus of open-heart surgery and coronary bypass, great strides were made in the quality of image amplification, particularly with the introduction of the cesium iodide tube. Simultaneously, powerful generators were developed, capable of millisecond exposures and high contrast levels. The cine cameras have evolved into dependable instruments with fine quality lens, so that the resolution of modern 35-mm cineangiocardiography is extraordinarily good. Video recording techniques have also improved strikingly. Instantaneous playback of tape-recorded images has afforded great utility and safety in determining whether the desired anatomic and physiologic information has been attained, thereby precluding additional unneccessary studies.

The most important technical innovation of the past few years has been the introduction of angled views to the study of congenital and acquired heart disease [8–11]. The equipment companies have responded to this innovation with engineering advances which have made angled views relatively simple. The 'C' arm, the 'U' arm, and the 'parallelogram' have all contributed

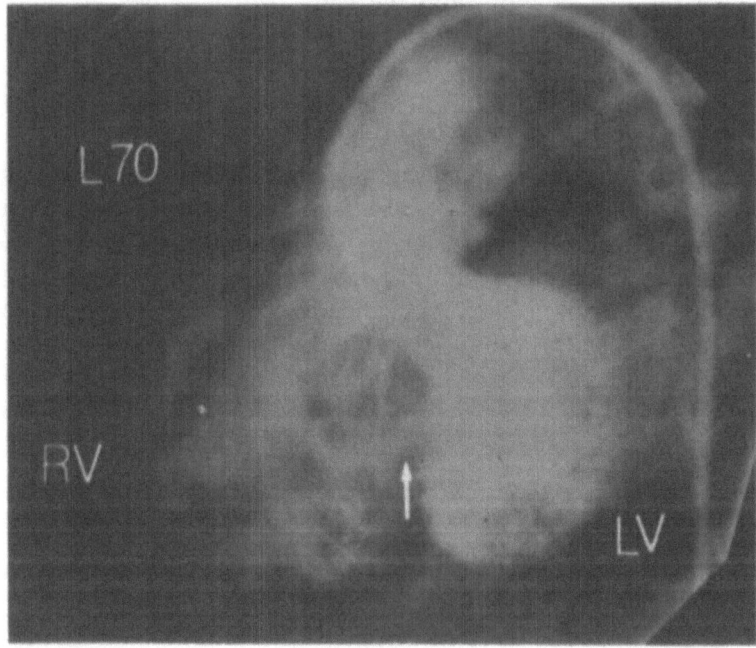

Fig. 1A. Ventricular septal defects. Injection has been made into the left ventricle via a catheter inserted through the aortic value. Conventional left anterior oblique projection, 70°. The left ventricle is opacified, and a shunt from left to right (arrow) produces corresponding opacification of the right ventricle. (Courtesy of Dr. Kenneth Fellows.)

immensely to our capacity to attain angled images without excessive time or patient movement.

Thus, they have been used to simplify and standardize angled views, although these can readily be accomplished with conventional equipment [8–11].

What have angled views accomplished? In congenital heart disease, they have enabled the separation of the four cardiac chambers and the delineation of the ventricular outflow tract and the interventricular septum never before definable with such clarity and precision. In such complex anomalies as endocardial cushion defects and double outlet right ventricle, virtually all elements of the deranged anatomy may now be demonstrated with great precision. In the tetralogy of Fallot, the pulmonary artery bifurcation is defined and the ventricular septum thrown into sharp relief, so that the size, position, and number of muscular ventricular septal defects are readily demonstrated (Fig. 1). In many other lesions – transposition, truncus, asymmetrical septal hypertrophy, subvalvular membranous aortic stenosis, etc. – angled views add enormously to the anatomic knowledge essential for appropriate diagnosis and treatment.

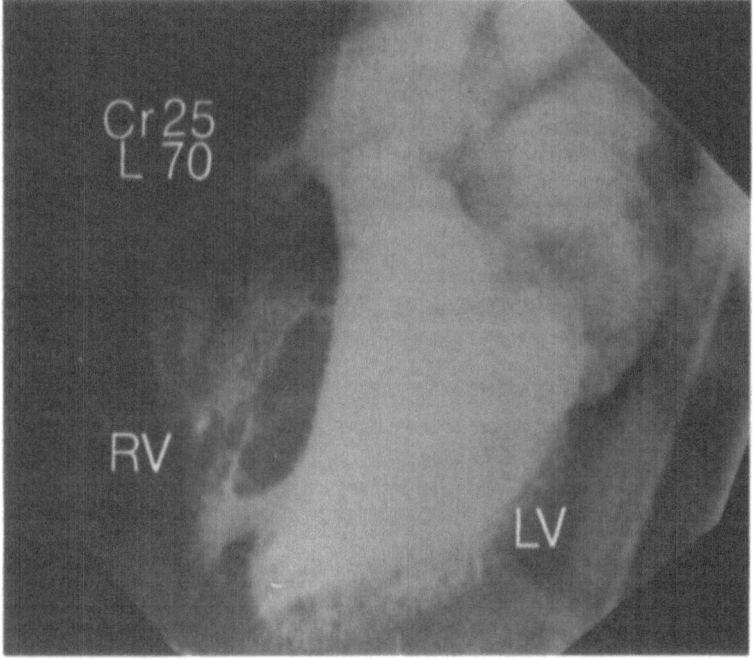

Fig. 1B. Ventricular septal defects. Injection has been made into the left ventricle via a catheter inserted through the aortic valve. Left anterior oblique projection, angled 25° cranially. The ventricular septum is now thrown into sharp relief, and three separate ventricular septal defects are visualized in the muscular septum. (Courtesy of Dr. Kenneth Fellows.)

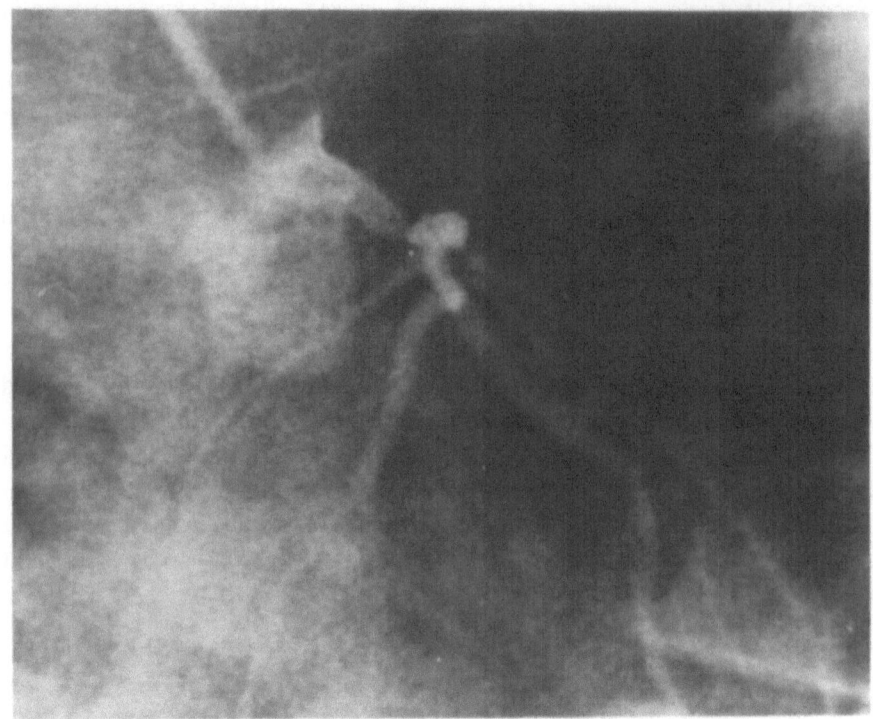

Fig. 2A. Coronary ateriography, left main coronary artery stenosis. Left anterior oblique projection, 60°. The left main coronary artery is well visualized, and there appears to be a moderate degree of stenosis just proximal to the bifurcation of the left anterior descending and circumflex arteries. The area is not well visualized.

Similarly, in the presence of suspected coronary artery disease, the angled views sometimes demonstrate highly significant stenosis either unsuspected or poorly visualized in conventional projections (Fig. 2).

QUALITATIVE VENTRICULOGRAPHY

A major advance in angiocardiography has involved the analysis of ventricular wall motion and behavior in coronary dissease from a qualitative point of view. In 1965, Harrison introduced the term 'asynergy' to describe the poor teamwork of the musculature of the left ventricle in some patients with coronary disease[12], and in 1967 the concept of asynergy was amplified[13, 14]. Four distinct types were described: akinesis, a total lack of motion of a portion of the left ventricular wall; asyneresis, diminished or inadequate motion of part of the wall; dyskinesis, paradoxical systolic expansion; and asynchrony, a disturbed temporal sequence of contraction[15]. Hypokinesis was reserved for a generalized reduction in left ventricular con-

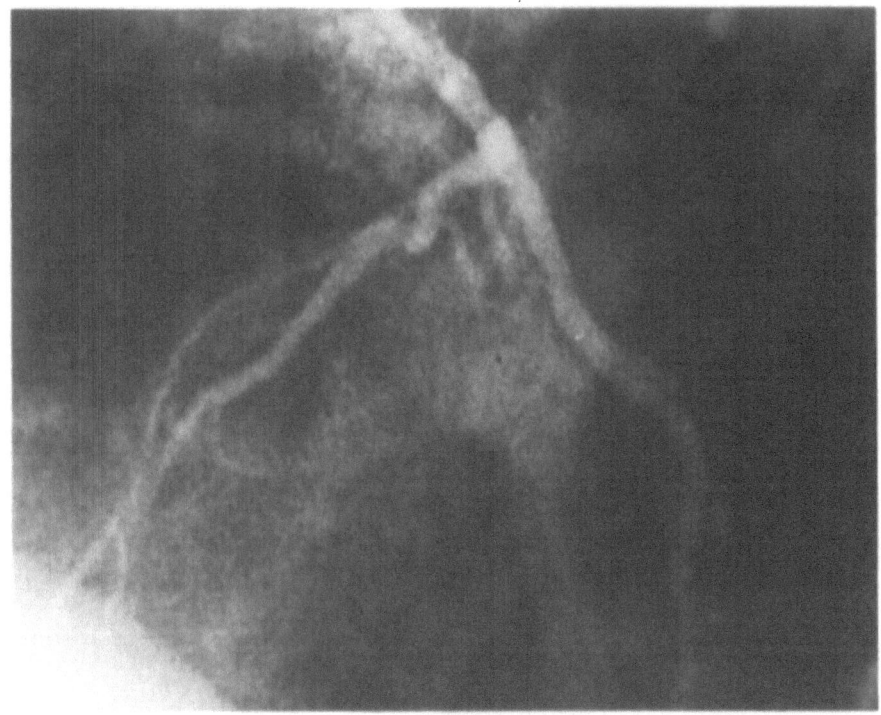

Fig. 2B. Coronary arteriography, left main coronary artery stenosis. Lateral projection. No definite evidence of left main coronary artery stenosis is seen. Multiple small plaques are visible along the length of the left anterior descending and circumflex arteries.

traction but, in general use, has now become interchangeable with asyneresis when the local area is specified (e.g., anterior wall hypokinesis).

Although common, the exact incidence of asynergy in ischemic heart disease is unknown. The patients who undergo ventriculography are preselected and, because an area of asynergy may be histologically normal, pathologic series are misleading. The following figures on incidence of asynergy are a rough guide: 52% in angina without prior infarction but with major disease in at least one vessel[16]; 79% in patients with acute myocardial infarction[17]; and 67%–76% in patients with previous myocardial infarction [17, 18].

The sites of asynergy can be consistently related to significant disease in the appropriate coronary artery[13, 19, 20]. Its prevalence increases with the number of vessels involved[21]. Areas of asynergy may be single or multiple, and on pathologic examination may show normal myocardium, fibrous replacement of muscle, complete or incomplete[15] or acute infarction. Even a ventriculographic aneurysm may show only scattered fibrosis in predominantly viable muscle[13].

125

Thus, asynergy may be due to replacement of myocardium by fibrosis or to a more subtle derangement in the contractile process.

After Harrison suggested that ventricular asynergy might be important in the genesis of cardiac failure in coronary artery disease [12], convincing supporting evidence was produced by subsequent workers [19]. An akinetic area of sufficient size may give rise to ventricular failure despite normal myocardium in the remainder of the ventricle. The therapeutic implication is that such areas may be surgically resectable or may be improved by successful aortocoronary saphenous vein bypass.

With the use of qualitative ventriculography, the definition of ventricular aneurysm has also changed. It is now variously described as 'a protusion of a localized portion of the external aspect of the left ventricle beyond the remainder of the cardiac surface, with simultaneous protrusion of the cavity as well' [22], a 'circumscribed outpouching of the left ventricle' [23], and an area of akinesis or dyskinesis [13]. The last definition includes cases in which akinesis or dyskinesis is seen in an area of viable myocardium and is thus a physiologic aneurysm [13]. Efforts have been made to differentiate the two on

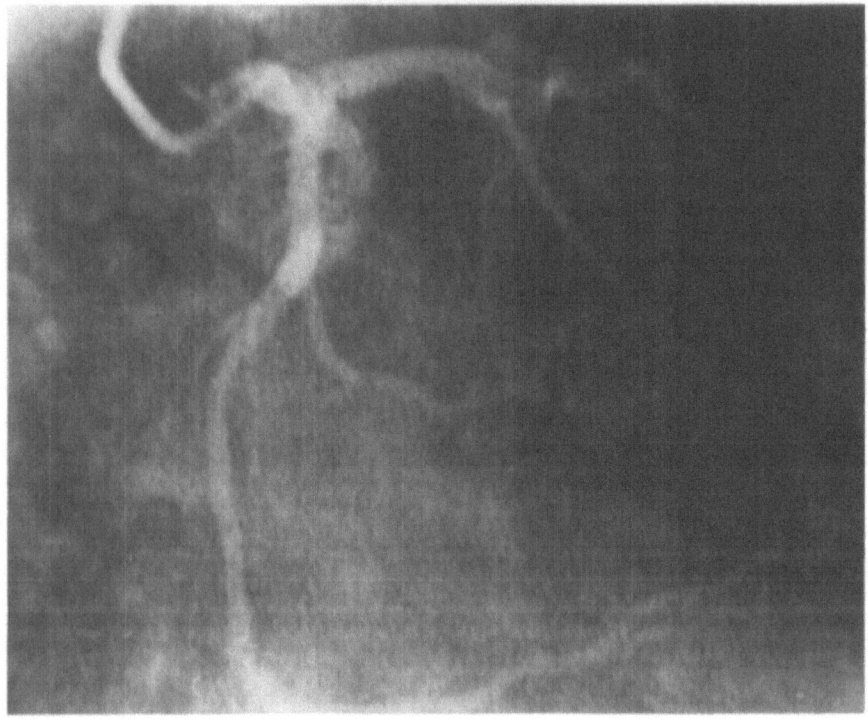

Fig. 2C. Coronary arteriography, left main coronary artery stenosis. Right anterior oblique projection. There is no evidence of significant stenosis of the left main, left anterior descending, or circumflex ateries.

angiographic criteria, mainly chamber size and extent of wall involvement [24]. The distinction is of major importance. An aneurysm in which total muscle destruction has occurred must be resected if it plays a role in cardiac failure by decreasing left ventricular efficiency. A functional aneurysm with viable muscle in its wall is probably best treated by revascularization.

In 1955, I made a prediction which I would like to quote verbatim:
As experience with angiocardiography has increased, it has become apparent that its pre-eminent role in diagnosis will relate to congenital cardiac anomalies rather than acquired heart disease. The reason for this inheres both in the nature of the disease and in the limitations of the technique. The age group in which congenital heart disease occurs is obviously much younger than that of acquired heart disease. Hence, the injected medium has a much shorter distance to traverse, remains in much higher concentration, and usually delineates chamber size, right-to-left shunts, valvular stenosis, and great vessel overriding with clarity. Many of the congenital anomalies in which angiocardiography is most useful involve the right heart chambers and can be diagnosed by right heart opacification alone.

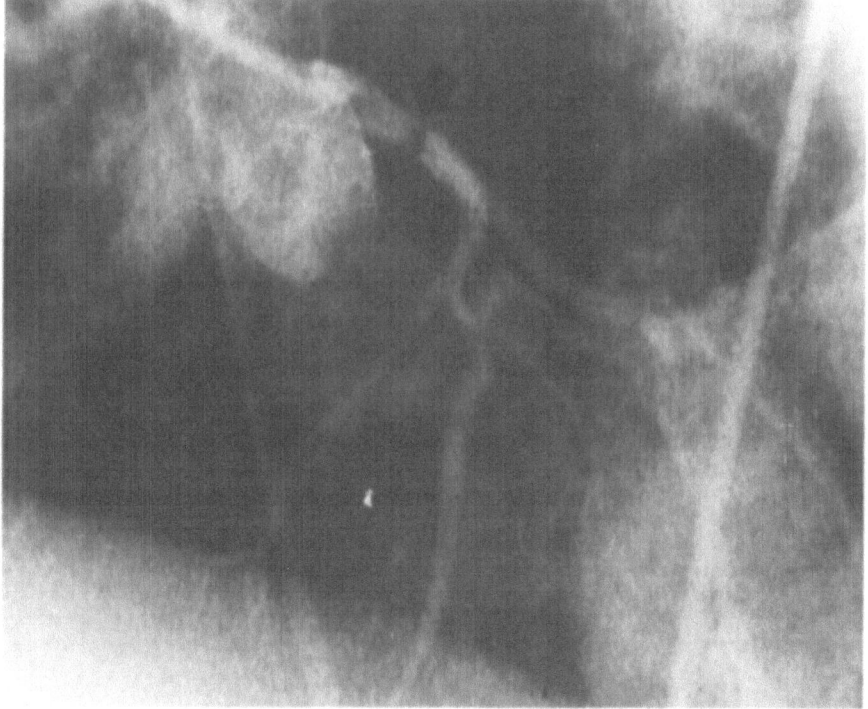

Fig. 2D. Coronary arteriography, left main coronary artery stenosis. Left anterior oblique projection, 70°, with cranial angulation of 30°. A very severe stenosis of the left main coronary artery is now clearly shown (arrow).

Conversely, most acquired heart disease affects the left heart or the entire heart, and frequently the myocardium is involved rather than the valves or the septa. [1]

This prediction has clearly been proved wrong by the march of technical events. Angiocardiography, in the modern era, has critically important applications to acquired heart disease and represents the most definitive approach to defining operable coronary disease and to the study of ventricular behavior in the presence of myocardial ischemia.

QUANTITATIVE VENTRICULOGRAPHY

Angiocardiography furnishes vital quantitative information related to ventricular function. As far back as 1956 and 1958, Dodge and Chapman perceived the potential of biplane ventriculography for furnishing data on ventricular volumes and stroke volumes, the one for large films [25], the other for cine [26]. Dodge refined the approaches to ventricular volume and emphasized the wide range of cardiodynamic data available from precisely synchronized studies [27]. Since that time, an extensive literature has accumulated on ventricular volumes, left ventricular wall mass, left ventricular compliance, work, power and the pressure volume loop, stroke volume, ejection fraction, velocity of fiber shortening, myocardial wall tension and stress, and myocardial hypertrophy [28]. These quantitative measurements have emphasized the interdependence of contrast visualization and pressure recording via the angiographic catheter that are so much a part of contemporary physiologic and clinical investigation. An exhaustive survey of their impact is beyond the scope of this review.

INTERVENTIONAL ANGIOCARDIOGRAPHY

One of the most dramatic of recent developments has been the application of the angiographic catheter to the nonoperative therapy of congenital and acquired heart disease. These advances have come about through the extraordinary ingenuity of a number of individuals who have utilized conventional catheter technology, refined it significantly, and demonstrated its value in specific applications.

Shunt closure

Patent ductus arteriosus. After experimental studies in animals, in 1971, Porstmann reported the use of the transfemoral approach to the closure of patent

128

ductus arteriosus in human subjects[29]. Closure was successful in 56 of 62 patients (90%); in two it was unsuccessful because the ductus was too small, and in four the procedure failed because the ductus was too large.

Kitamura in 1976 reported a group of 87 patients with transfemoral closure compared with a group of 100 who had surgical closure[30]. Complications occurred in 6% of the transfemoral closure group and in 14% of the surgical closure group.

Since his first report, Porstmann has attained nonsurgical ductal closure in a much larger series of patients, with the same degree of success demonstrated in the initial series. These youngsters are, therefore, spared the trauma of thoracotomy and surgery, and obtain a therapeutic result of equivalent quality in most cases.

Atrial septal defect. Within recent years, Rashkind has developed a transcatheter method of closing atrial septal defects[31]. The device includes an external catheter sheath, an internal catheter, a stainless-steel spring-wound guidewire, and a prosthesis consisting of a stainless-steel skeleton with a central cylindrical hub. Three arms are added into the hub and a disc of medical foam is used as a covering for the skeleton. The system resembles a 'miniaturized umbrella,' collapsed within the external carrying catheter. It has been applied to ten children with secundum atrial septal defects, with complete closure in six, satisfactory closure in three, and inadequate closure in one.

Ventricular septal defects. Thus far, transcatheter nonsurgical closure of ventricular septal defects has been performed in only the experimental animal[32]. The technology is advancing, however, and may soon be applicable to human subjects.

Shunt production

In 1966, Rashkind presented a preliminary communication reporting the results in seven puppies and in three infants with transposition of the great vessels of the production of atrial septal defects by 'balloon atrial septostomy'[33].

Surado in 1968 also demonstrated that the procedure could be done successfully, applying it to five patients with total anomalous pulmonary venous connection, in four of whom it was successful[34]. In 1971, Rashkind summarized his experience with balloon atrial septostomy in 135 patients with a variety of congenital heart lesions[35]. Among the 135, the septostomy was adequate in 129. It was most effective in transposition of the great vessels, tricuspid atresia, and total anomalous pulmonary venous return. Others have not been able to duplicate the high success rate that Rashkind has reported [36].

Dilatation of stenosed vessels and valves

Angioplasty in arteriosclerosis. Dotter and Judkins first reported the use of the catheter as a means of dilating narrowed blood vessels in man [37], and the Dotter technique of transluminal dilatation has now been widely applied, more in Europe than in the United States. Gruntzig modified the method to develop a balloon technology in 1977 and 1978, and recently has reported his results with a series of patients with coronary disease [38]. There is little question but that balloon dilatation in carefully chosen patients is successful in dilating narrowed coronary arteries and reducing pressure gradients. The method has now been applied to the renal arteries in the presence of hypertension with great success [39], and shows promise of being applicable to a number of visceral arteries. Its major application unquestionably is to ileofemoral and distal limb disease in which many reports of successful angioplasty are now available.

Coartation of the aorta. The successful application of balloon angioplasty to dysplastic disease of the renal arteries suggested the possibility that it might also be applicable to coarctation of the aorta. This has now been accomplished and a nonoperative approach to infants with significant coarctation is therefore now available [40].

Pulmonary valvotomy. A recent report has made clear the feasibility of non-surgical balloon catheter valvotomy [41]. In the presence of valvular pulmonic stenosis and heart failure, the valve was successfully dilated and the patient made an uneventful recovery. It is not yet clear how wide an application this method will have in valvular disease.

It is apparent, however, that we are now at the very beginning of a period during which the angiographic catheter may be increasingly employed for therapeutic approaches in heart disease as it has long been used for diagnosis.

THE POTENTIAL OF CARDIAC COMPUTED TOMOGRAPHY

The diagnosis of acute myocardial infarction is usually made on the basis of the clinical symptoms and signs, and corroborated by electrocardiography.

The effect of acute infarction depends on the amount of muscle tissue destroyed and the residual capacity of the left ventricle to accomplish its pumping functions efficiently. Within the last few years, a major effort has been initiated to intervene following infarction either pharmacologically or mechanically, with the specific objective of preserving viable but ischemic myocardium, and minimizing the volume of muscle lost. This effort has been limited by an incapacity to visualize the volume of infarcted myocardium with precision. The research in progress has depended on indirect methods to evaluate the impact of pharmacologic agents. The most useful direct approach employs radionuclides, a method limited by both image resolution and heterogeneous tissue uptake of the isotope.

In another critically important area of cardiac diagnosis, namely visualization of the interior of the cardiac chambers, we have relied until recently on invasive intracardiac catheterization and the rapid delivery of an iodinated contrast agent, recorded serially on cine or large film. Noninvasive techniques, such as radionuclide imaging and echocardiography have recently made great strides in becoming reproducible, dependable methods, but have significant limitations in resolution and extent of visualization.

Because of the central importance of these major areas of cardiac diagnosis, the potential usefulness of cardiac CT scanning is now under investigation. Initial studies focused on animal models in which a number of questions were asked:

1) Does infarcted myocardium have an attenuation coefficient sufficiently different from that of normal myocardium so that it can be visualized?
2) Can the interface between the intracardiac or intraventricular blood pool and the ventricular wall be delineated?
3) What is the role of contrast enhancement?
4) How do changes in myocardial attenuation coefficient correlate with blood flow?

Our earlier studies demonstrated that myocardium served by an artery which had been occluded experimentally developed a lower attenuation coefficient and therefore was visible as an area of relative lucency compared with normal myocardium [42, 43]. While the interface between the ventricular wall and the cavity was not distinguishable at normal hematocrit, it could readily be defined with lower hematocrit or with contrast enhancement. Furthermore, following coronary occlusion, the use of intravenous contrast agents enabled the visualization of the area of ischemia with great precision in studies in vitro of the dog heart. A good correlation was shown between diminution in blood flow as measured by microspheres and changes in myocardial attenuation coefficients [44]. It has also been shown that there is differential concentration of the contrast material in the infarcted area compared with normal myocardium [45, 46].

The application of data derived from both in vitro and in vivo animal studies to man was limited by the length of the scan time in the early CT units. With the development of faster scan times, it has become apparent that areas of myocardial thinning are demonstrable in human subjects, and that the cavity-wall interface can readily be distinguished by using contrast enhancement. The patency of coronary bypass graphs may be determined [46]. Both with and without gating to the electrocardiogram, it is apparent that cardiac computed tomography can be accomplished with the present level of technology [47, 48].

The potential of this method lies in the following areas:

1) A new approach to experimental study of tissue ischemia, infarction, and necrosis.
2) Detection, sizing, and dating of acute myocardial infarctions and the evaluation of the effectiveness of mechanical and pharmacological interventions designed to limit infarct size.
3) Evaluation of regional ventricular wall motion and thickness in acute and chronic myocardial ischemia.
4) Overall assessment of ventricular function through measurement of ventricular volumes, ejection fractions, and other physiologic parameters.
5) The detection of patency of coronary bypass grafts without invasive examination.
6) The assessment of obstructive cardiomyopathy, intracardiac tumors, and other forms of congenital and acquired heart disease noninvasively.
7) The detection, quantitation, and categorization of pericardial abnormalities, including effusion, pericardial tumors, cysts, and fat pads.

This discussion has focused on transmission cardiac tomography because it represents a form of roentgen contrast imaging of the cardiovascular system, or angiocardiography. It must also be emphasized that rapid strides are being made in emission computed tomography, which will equally provide important information about the condition of the myocardium and the cardiac chambers [49].

CONCLUSION

What will be the effect of the new imaging technologies – nuclear radiology, ultrasound, and computed tomography – on angiocardiography? There will surely be a decreased need for ventriculography and for invasive follow-up examinations in postsurgical patients. But is seems likely that for many years to come all potential candidates for cardiac surgery – coronary, valvular, and congenital – will remain proper subjects for meticulous angiocardiographic examinations. No other method affords the extraordinary resolution now available. The surgeon requires a precise and accurate roadmap if operating time is to be minimized and successful correction maximized; to this end, angiocardiography comprises the 'gold standard' for the study of all forms of congenital and acquired heart disease.

REFERENCES

1. Abrams HL, Kaplan HS (1956) Angiocardiographic interpretation in congenital heart disease. Springfield IL: Charles C Thomas
2. Abrams HL (1955) Radiologic aspects of operable heart disease. I. Observations on the preoperative approach to congenital anomalies. Radiology 65:31–49
3. Abrams HL (1956) Radiologic aspects of operable heart disease. II. Retrograde brachial aortography. Circulation 14:593–613
4. Heinz R, Abrams HL (1957) Radiologic aspects of operable heart disease. IV. The variable appearance of constrictive pericarditis. Radiology 69:54–62
5. Abrams HL (1957) Radiologic aspects of operable heart disease. V. The appearance of coarctation of the aorta in infancy. Stanford Med Bull 15:233–241
6. Strauss P, Abrams HL, Robinson S (1958) Radiologic aspects of operable heart disease. VI. Changes following surgical closure of patent ductus arteriosus. Circulation 17:1047–1055
7. Abrams HL (1959) An approach to biplane cineangiocardiography. III. Early clinical observations. Radiology 73: 531–538
8. Bargeron LM, Elliott LP, Soto B, Bream PR, Curry GC (1977) Axial cineangiography in congenital heart disease. I. Concept, technical and anatomic considerations. Circulation 56:1075–1083
9. Elliott LP, Bargeron LM, Bream PR, Soto B, Curry GC (1975) Axial cineangiography in congenital heart disease. II. Specific lesions. Circulation 56:1084–1093
10. Sos TA, Lee VG, Levin DC, Baltaxe HA (1974) New lordotic projection for improved visualization of the left coronary artery and its branches. Am J Roentgen Ray 121:575
11. Bunnell IL, Greene DG, Tandon RN, Arani DT (1973) The half-axial projection. A new look at the proximal left coronary artery. Circulation 48:1151
12. Harrison TR (1965) Some unanswered questions concerning enlargement and failure of the heart. Am Heart J 69:100
13. Gorlin R, Klein MD, Sullivan JM (1967) Prospective correlative study of ventricular aneurysm: mechanistic concept and clinical recognition. Am J Med 42:512
14. Herman MV, Gorlin R (1969) Implications of left ventricular asynergy. Am J Cardiol 23:538; Semin Roentgenol 4:346
15. Herman MV, Heinle RA, Klein MD, Gorlin R (1967) Localized disorders in myocardial contraction: asynergy and its role in congestive heart failure. N Engl J Med 277:222
16. Bjork L, Cullhed I, Hallen A (1967) Cineangiocardiographic studies of the left ventrical in patients with angina pectoris. Circulation 36:868
17. Kazamias TM, Gander MP, Ross J, Braunwald E (1971) Detection of left ventricular-wall motion disorders in coronary-artery disease by radarkymography. N Engl J Med 285:63
18. Baxley WA, Reeves TJ (1971) Abnormal regional myocardial performance in coronary artery disease. Prog Cardiovasc Dis 13:405

133

19. Herman MV, Gorlin R (1969) Implications of left ventricular asynergy. Am J Cardiol 23:538; Semin Roentgenol 4:346
20. McConahay DR, McCallister BD, Hallermann FJ, Smith RE (1970) Comparative quantitative analysis of the electrocardiogram and vectorcardiogram: correlation with the coronary arteriogram. Circulation 42:245
21. Helfant RH, Kemp HG, Gorlin R (1970) Coronary atherosclerosis, coronary collaterals, and their relation to cardiac function. Ann Intern Med 73:189
22. Edwards JE (1961) An atlas of acquired diseases of the heart and great vessels, vol 2. Philadelphia: Saunders
23. Abrams DL, Edelist A, Luria MH, Miller AJ (1963) Ventricular aneurysm: a reappraisal based on a study of sixty-five consecutive autopsied cases. Circulation 27:164
24. Raphael MJ, Steiner RE, Goodwin JF, Oakley CM (1972) Cine angiography of left ventricular aneurysms. Clin Radiol 23:129
25. Dodge HT, Tennenbaum HL (1956) Left ventricular volume in normal man and alterations with disease. Circulation 14:927
26. Chapman CB, Baker O, Reynolds J, Bonte FJ (1958) Use of biplane cinefluorography for measurement of ventricular volume. Circulation 18:1105
27. Dodge HT, Sandler H, Baxley WA, Hawley RR (1966) Usefulness and limitations of radiographic methods for determining left ventricular volume. Am J Cardiol 18:10
28. Moseley RD, Baker DH, Gorson RO, Lalli A, Latourette HB, Quinn JL (1974) Current problems in radiology; angiocardiographic quantitation of ventricular volume, shape and mass, vol 4.
29. Porstmann W, Wierney L, Warnke H, Gerstberger G, Romaniuk PA (1971) Catheter closure of patent ductus arteriosus; 62 cases treated without thoracotomy. Radiol Clin North Am IX. 2:203
30. Kitamura S, Sato K, Naito Y, Shimizu Y, Fujino M, Oyama C, Nakano S, Kawashima Y (1976) Plug closure of patent ductus arteriosus by transfemoral catheter method. Chest 70:631
31. Rashkind W (1978) Transcatheter closure of atrial septal defects program. Pediatr Radiol 7, Nr 6 C
32. Rashkind W (1979) Personal communication, 3 October
33. Rashkind W, Miller W (1966) Creation of an atrial septal defect without thoracotomy; a palliative approach to complete transposition of the great arteries. JAMA 196:173
34. Serratto M, Buchcleres HG, Bicoff P, Miller RA, Hastreiter AR (1968) Palliative balloon atrial septostomy for total anomalous pulmonary venous connection in infancy. J Pediatr 5:734–739
35. Rashkind W (1971) Atriospetostomy by balloon catheter in congenital heart disease. Radiol Clin North Am IX. 2:193
36. Hawker RE, Krovetz LJ, Rowe RD (1974) An analysis of prognostic factors in the outcome of balloon atrial septostomy for transposition of the great arteries. Johns Hopkins Med J 134:95–106
37. Dotter CT, Judkins MP (1964) Transluminal treatment of arteriosclerotic obstruction: description of a new technic and a preliminary report of its application. Circulation 30:654–670
38. Gruntzig AR, Senning A, Siegenthaler WE (1979 Nonoperative dilatation of coronary-artery stenosis. N Engl J Med 301:61–68
39. Millan VG, Mast WE, Madias NE (1979) Nonsurgical treatment of severe hypertension due to renal-artery intimal fibroplasia by percutaneous transluminal angioplasty. N Engl J Med 300:1371–1373
40. Sos T: Personal communications

41. Semb BKH, Tjonneland S, Stake G, Aabyholm G (1979) Balloon valvulotomy of congenital pulmonary valve stenosis with tricuspid valve insufficiency. Cardiovasc Radiol 2:239

42. Adams D, Hessel SJ, Judy PF, Stein JA, Abrams HL (1976) Differing attenuation coefficients of normal and infarcted myocardium. Science 192:467–469

43. Adams D, Hessel SJ, Judy PF, Stein JA, Abrams HL (1976) Computed tomography of the normal and infarcted myocardium. Am J Roentgenol 126:786–791

44. Hessel SJ, Adams D, Judy PF, et al. (1978) Detection of myocardial ischemia in vitro by computed tomography. Radiology 127:413

45. Carlsson E, Lipton MJ, Berninger WH, et al. (1977) Selective left coronary myocardiography by computed tomography in living dogs. Invest Radiol 12:559

46. Higgins CB, Schmidt W, Siemers PT, et al. (1979) Evaluation of myocardial ischemic damage of varying ages by computerized transmission tomography. Time dependent effects of contrast material. Circulation 60:284

47. Guthaner DF, Brody WR, Ricci M, Oyer PE, Wexler L (1979) The use of computed tomography in the diagnosis of coronary artery bypass graft patency. Cardiovasc Radiol 3:2–6

48. Moncada R, Churchill R, Reynes C, Love L, Hale DJ, Schreiber R, Matias S (1979) CT of the pericardium, heart and coronaries. Presented at the 65th annual meeting of the Radiologic Society of North America, Atlanta, 25–30 November

49. Zielonka JS, Holman BL (1979) Emission tomography of the heart: principles and applications. Cardiovasc Radiol 2:217

PART THREE

History of cardiac surgery

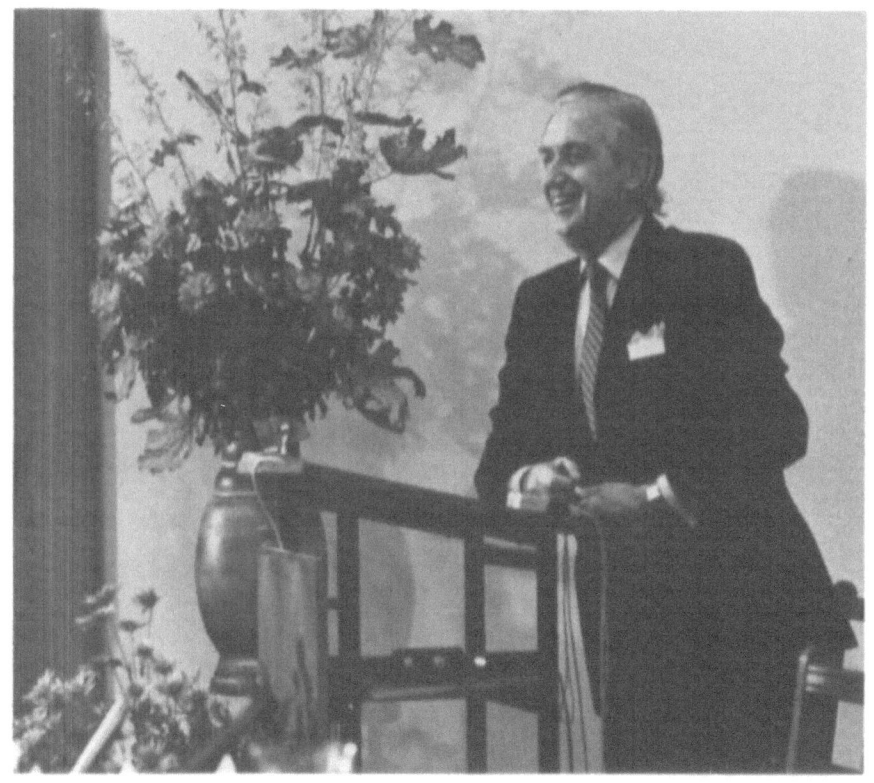

Dr. A. G. Brom, chairman of the session.

HENRY SWAN

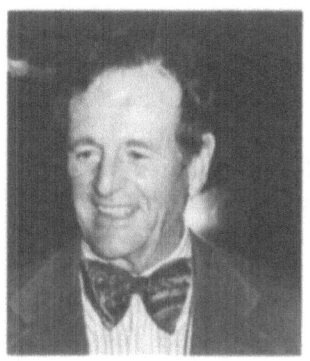

Dr. Henry Swan, born in 1913, is surgeon at the Colorado General Hospital in Denver, Colorado, and clinical professor of surgery and surgical research at the University of Colorado's School of Medicine. He has made major contributions in vascular research and toward hypothermia in the surgical treatment of arterial vessel disease.

Cardiac surgery with hypothermia

It is an honor for me to have been asked to give the opening lecture in this symposium on the history of heart surgery. I shall attempt to describe the prolonged growing-pains of direct cardiac intervention and to discuss the part hypothermia has played in opening the interior of the heart to operative repair. Hypothermia was the method which broke the barrier to the inner recesses of the heart as the proper domain of the surgeon; hypothermia remains today as the keystone of all successful techniques to preserve that right of eminent domain. I shall try to highlight this story for you succinctly.

You see, the heart was the last organ of the body to enter the happy realm of reparative surgery. Its debut was marked by defiance of sacred belief and was clothed in dire prophecies of failure. Already by 1890 the abdomen had succumbed to the ovariotomists, and the neurosurgeons were resurrecting what was perhaps the oldest surgical invasion of a body cavity – trephining the skull. Anesthesia from America had been endorsed by the Queen of England, and Pasteur and Lister had led the way to antisepsis.

But mythology held a firm grip on the imagination of the medical profession and the people as a whole. The heart was considered the seat of the soul; it was known to be 'a delicate organ which succumbed to the slightest injury.' These ideas had prevailed for centuries. Thus, wounds of the heart had been treated only by removal of the penetrating weapon; no other procedures were tried. It is understandable why the great Theodor Billroth proclaimed in 1895 in no uncertain terms that the surgeon who would presume to operate deliberately upon the heart would lose the respect of all his colleagues and should be banished from the practice of his profession.

139

As if to prove him wrong, the very next year at the Surgical Congress in Rome, the young Italian surgeon del Vecchio displayed live on the stage three dogs in whom he had made an incision through the muscle of the ventricle which he had closed by suture with linen thread. The playful activity of the dogs left no doubt as to the successful outcome of this operation upon the very muscle of the heart itself. Among those sitting in that distinguished audience was Ludwig Rehn of Frankfurt. Within the year, the first major event in heart surgery occurred. Rehn accomplished the first successful suture of a wound of the human heart. Reparative surgery of the injured heart was off to a shaky start which nevertheless in the next two decades resulted in widespread understanding and management of pericardial tamponade, together with suture closure of lacerations of auricle and ventricle.

In the laboratories, men of vision, imagination, and daring began to solve the techniques of cardiovascular surgery. In his remarkable book published in 1905, Benjamin Ricketts described experimental suture of ventricular wounds in dogs, and gave an exhaustive review of the world literature on cardiac surgery to that date. Alexis Carrel, transplanted from Lyon to Chicago to New York's Rockefeller Institute, solved the problems of vascular suture, arterial grafting, and the transplantation of organs. In addition, he studied methods to operate upon the aortic and pulmonary valves, which he presented to the American Surgical Society in 1914 in a remarkable address. Meanwhile, Haecker in Germany had demonstrated the merits of temporary venous inflow occlusion as a means for intracardiac manipulation. And in 1913, E. Jeger published his remarkable book *Surgery of the Blood Vessels and Heart*. In it are demonstrated essentially all of the techniques of vascular suture and grafting, of cardiac incisions and their repair, and of intracardiac manipulation during inflow occlusion by using appropriate noncrushing clamps. In this book is shown an explicit illustration of a technique to bypass a stenotic aortic valve by using a venous graft with its intrinsic values – a technique rediscovered by Sarnoff and others 40 years later? And do you suppose Dr. Blalock would have blushed to see aortopulmonary diversion precisely decribed 30 years before his time?

So by 1913 it was clear that the surgical techniques to operate upon the heart were developed to a point where deliberate attack upon the morpholog- ical lesions of congenital, valvular, or atherosclerotic heart disease was feasi- ble. Why were they not applied clinically? Meltzer and Auer had already published in 1909 the secret of intratracheal positive pressure, and in 1911 Elsberg had given the first clinical anesthesia for open-chest surgery. More- over, after World War I, Russia and the Balkan countries developed blood banking: Yudin is one of the fathers of blood transfusion. So surgery of the heart, which had needed the stepping stones of (a) the conquest of surgery of the open chest and (b) of blood transfusion, before it could be admitted to the operating rooms of the Western World, was ready. But even so, mythology and the spectre of Billroth still stood forebodingly in the doorway.

It was within this context that the second major event in the story of heart surgery took place in 1938. The primary credit must really go to a pediatrician. Dr. John Hubbard in Boston referred for surgery a healthy, symptom-free eight-year-old girl with patent ductus. Thus, Robert E. Gross was given the opportunity to challenge the prejudice of the ages. His patient, a little girl, left Boston Children's Hospital on the 10th postoperative day, cured of her congenital heart disease. Neither cardiology nor cardiac surgery has ever been the same since that day. Surgery had been ready, but it was John Hubbard who had had the courage to refer the right patient! I was fortunate enough to have been the medical student helping at surgery on this child; an event which no doubt influenced my own future role in surgery of the heart.

So now the gauntlet was on the ground at the feet of pediatricians and cardiologists alike around the world. Before Hubbard and Gross, the precise diagnosis of congenital heart disease was seldom achieved; indeed it was seldom attempted. Since there was, up to that time, no significant means to improve the prognosis of kids with murmurs or of blue babies, why bother with definitive workups? But now it was clear there was *one* form of congenital heart disease which could be cured by surgery. The challenge was frontal; at least patent ductus arteriosus must be distinguished from all others, so that the patient must be offered a cure. Dr. Dexter described yesterday how cardiology jumped to meet this challenge by the surgeon. Keener clinical evaluation, better fluoroscopy and radiology, cardiac catheterization, pressure transducers and oxymeters, and improved electrocardiography soon led to rapidly expanding precision in preoperative diagnosis and postoperative evaluation in congenital heart disease. Dr. Einthoven, from his view on high, must have beamed with pleasure to witness the flowering of his techniques in the exciting decades following his death.

But, then again, the world tied itself up in global war, and elective surgery of the heart had to wait. Thus, it was that the postwar decade between 1944 and 1953 became the era of pericardiac and closed-heart manipulative techniques. Resection of coarctation of the aorta, developed by Crafoord and Gross, and the aortopulmonary anastamoses of Blalock and Potts added importantly to the list of curable or remedial congenital heart disease, although the procedures were not really performed on the heart itself but on the great vessels surrounding it. Now *all* the various forms of both acyanotic and cyanotic heart disease had to be identified.

To help in this challenge, emerged the most respected, influential, and beloved pediatric cardiologist of the era, indeed probably of all time, Helen Taussig. Her monumental work, *Congenital Malformations of the Heart,* codified and correlated pathologic anatomy with the distortions in circulation, and defined the nature of the changing pathophysiology, as misdirection and volume of flow progressed. The worlds of cardiology and cardiac surgery can never express adequately their debt of gratitude for guidance at this moment in medical history to this remarkable 'Lady of the Heart' whom we are privileged to have here with us, and who will honor us by her reminiscences later this morning.

As for surgery within the heart itself, this was the era of skilled blind manipulation with finger or instrument inserted via ventricle or auricular appendage, with hemorrhage controlled by purse-string suture. The transventricular incision of the stenotic pulmonary valve first performed by Sellors, later extensively developed by Brock and others, using graded knives or the expanding knife of Potts and instrumental dilatation of the stenotic mitral valve, was increasingly performed.

Who can forget Harkens and Bailey holding forth simultaneously in passionate defence of 'commissurotomy' versus 'valvuloplasty' in front of their rival exhibits at thoracic surgical meetings in the closing years of the 1940s? And at the beginning of the 1950s, Andrew Logan and Charles Dubost's power-dilators increased the enlargement of leathery or stony valves. Even auricular septal defects were closed under digital guidance by Søndergaard's encircling suture, Bailey's atrioseptopexy, or via the Gross well.

True, sometimes serious regurgitations or peripheral embolization occurred following these closed mitral procedures; and there was a steady recurrence rate of stenosis with the passage of time. But let us not forget also that these procedures were done at less than a tenth the cost to the patient of modern cardiac bypass surgery, and that many patients were completely free of symptoms for periods measured by decades. Who among us would confidently predict how many satisfactory 20-, 25-, and even 30-year follow-ups we shall see in patients with artificial heart valves? Ultraexpensive modern surgery just may *not* be the best answer in every patient.

Surgical attack upon organic abnormalities of the heart came to be accepted more and more during this period. The ghost of Billroth was finally being laid to rest. Surgeons had learned to combat the terrors of cardiac arrest and acute fibrillatory emergencies. Claude Beck had pled successfully at last for resuscitation of hearts 'too good to die.' The techniques of closed cardiac and vascular surgery, anesthesia for the open chest, blood transfusion, antibiotics and, perhaps most important, *acceptance of the idea of heart surgery* were at last all in place.

But how to get sufficient time to operate within the opened heart remained, in 1950, the piece necessary to complete the puzzle. At this moment in time, April of 1950, a paper was presented at the meeting of the American Surgical Association in Colorado Springs, Colorado. Wilfried Bigelow of Toronto described how he had cooled anesthetized dogs in ice water to a rectal temperature of 20°–25°C, had then stopped their body circulation by vena caval occlusion for 15 minutes, and after that had rewarmed the dogs until they were breathing spontaneously. He remarked that since these were not primarily survival experiments, 85% of the dogs succumbed to the procedure; but he noted that the surviving dogs were normal in every way, showing no evidence of brain damage or other organ–system injury. I heard a prominent gastric surgeon remark to his companion: 'Say, that hypothermia is really dangerous; I'm going to get a better overcoat.' But, driving home to Denver the next day, I was thinking about Dr. Bigelow's stimulating report when suddenly its message sank home to me. It wasn't the 85% mortality rate; the fact was *that 15% of the hypothermic animals had survived total cessation of circulation for 15 minutes, a period of time which would be universally fatal at a normal body temperature.* What needed to be done was to learn to control the parameters of risk associated with body cooling in order to achieve that wonderful 15 minutes for operation within the open heart! Within the week, my research grant application was in the mail to Bethesda, and the Halsted Laboratory of Surgical Research at the University of Colorado had already cooled its first dog in ice water. A year and a half and over 400 dogs later, we felt ready to try our first human case. Several more followed rapidly and in June of 1953 the report of the first successful series of patients with various forms of intracardiac congenital anomalies undergoing corrective surgery *by direct vision in the open heart* was published. Since there was only one death among these 13 patients, this publication proved decisively that a means had at last been found to operate safely *within* the heart. Thus, at long last, the heart entered the company of all the other organs as being a proper subject for surgical correction.

This emphasizes what I think is one of the unique and remarkable aspects of the development of cardiac surgery compared with other anatomic forms of surgery. Unlike abdominal, central nervous system, or pulmonary surgery (for example), all of which were developed by experience gained primarily in the human operating room and subsequent necropsy, surgery of the heart was first learned, and the early tentative mistakes were made, in the experimental laboratory. I have mentioned that over 400 dog experiments antedated our first human case; some sense of mastery over the dreaded complications of hypothermia, namely, ventricular fibrillation and bleeding dyscrasias, had already been published.

Simultaneously, and subsequently, Bigelow, Zindler, Lewis, Sealy and Brown, Brock, Julian, Brom, Husfeldt, Dubost, Shumacker, Lam, Valdoni, Scott, Boerema, and many others were vigorously exploring the management of various operative techniques during cooling. Thus, from the very first, heart surgery was associated with low operative mortality rates. For example, our first 69 patients with isolated pulmonary valvular stenosis, beginning with patient one, were operated on without a single postoperative death, and by 1955 open repair of atrial septal defect during hypothermia carried less operative risk than resection of the gall bladder (Fig. 1).

Open heart procedures using hypothermia alone

Disease	Patients	Deaths
I.A.S.D., Secundum	205	10
Pulm. valv. stenosis	69	0
Pulm. infund. stenosis	10	1
Trilogy of fallot	31	5
Tetralogy of fallot	19	2
Pentalogy of fallot	3	1
Aortic valvular stenosis	34	2
Aortic subvalvular stenosis	6	5
	377	26 (6.8%)

Fig. 1. Results of early operative experience using hypothermia at Colorado Medical Center were published in 1958.

Some of the various techniques to induce hypothermia involved surface cooling, others used some form of perfusion, and Charles Hufnagel developed local cooling of the heart in ice chips, a technique still widely used today. Our own technique was rapid and reasonably controllable. The patient was first anesthetized with ether and then immersed in a large tub of ice water (Fig. 2). This tub, like Dr. Burch's space-flying monkey 'Able,' now resides in the Smithsonian Institute in Washington. To protect against ventricular fibrillation, we used various steps to achieve a stable level of body temperature at 30 °C. Time and cryophysiology have now proven that our insistence upon hyperventillation to achieve a high pH was the correct way to achieve biological hydroxyl hydrogen ion ratios at low temperature.

Using this methodology for a broad variety of open-heart procedures, we were able to report these overall results at about the time when the cardiopulmonary bypass machines were becoming available for intracardiac procedures.

At the end of this era, in 1958, with the increasing adoption of various 'heart–lung machines' as they were then called, heart surgery could turn to new methodologies. At first bypass was used *instead* of hypothermia. Indeed, one well-known Texas surgeon joined Billroth as an example of how poor surgeons can be as prophets – he was busy trying to organize 'The Society for the Prevention of Hypothermia.' But soon the advantages of combining mild hypothermia with perfusion became apparent and it was not long until, at the

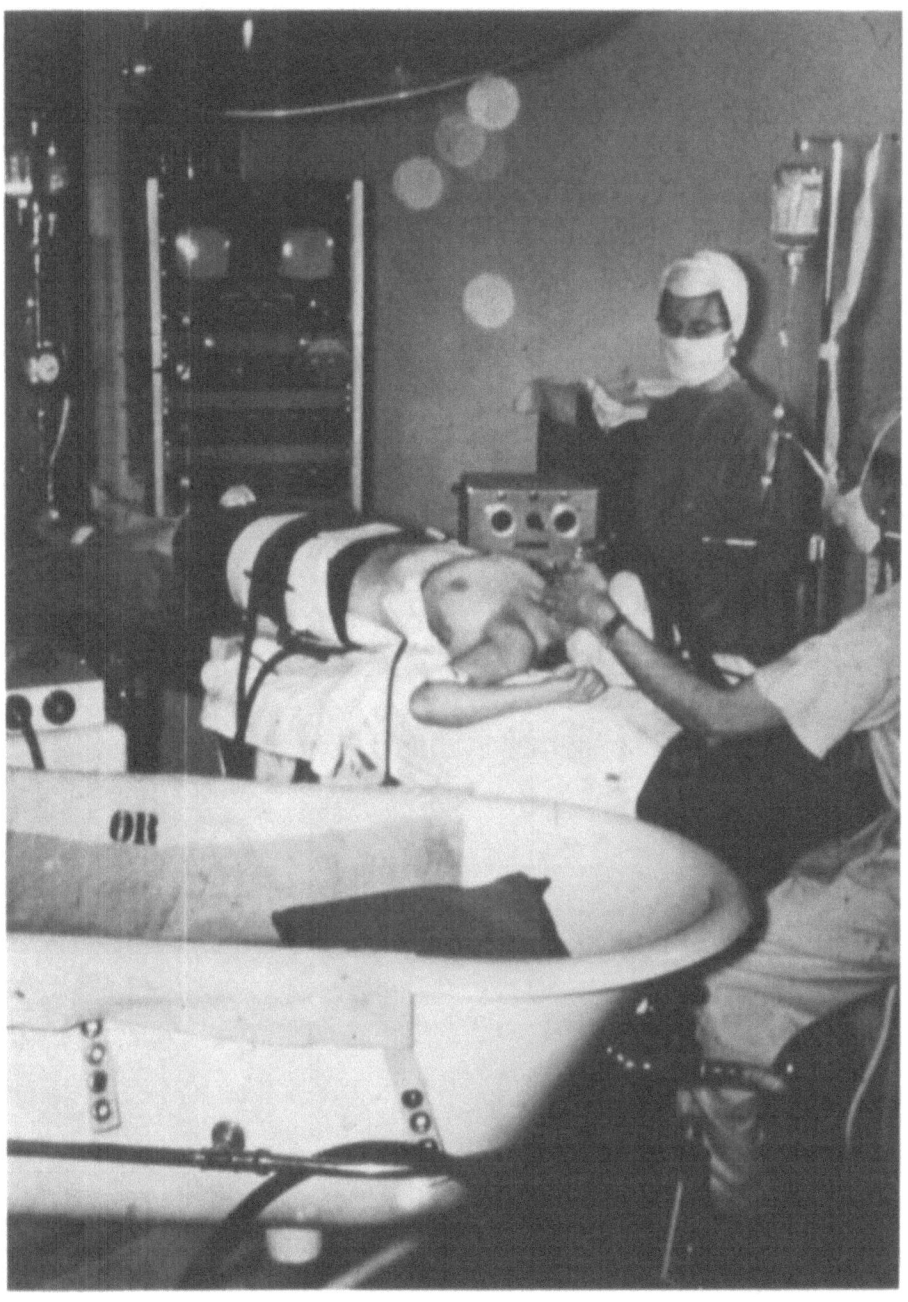

Fig. 2. Immersion cooling in ice water and rewarming with diathermy was the standard management of clinical hypothermia at Colorado.

145

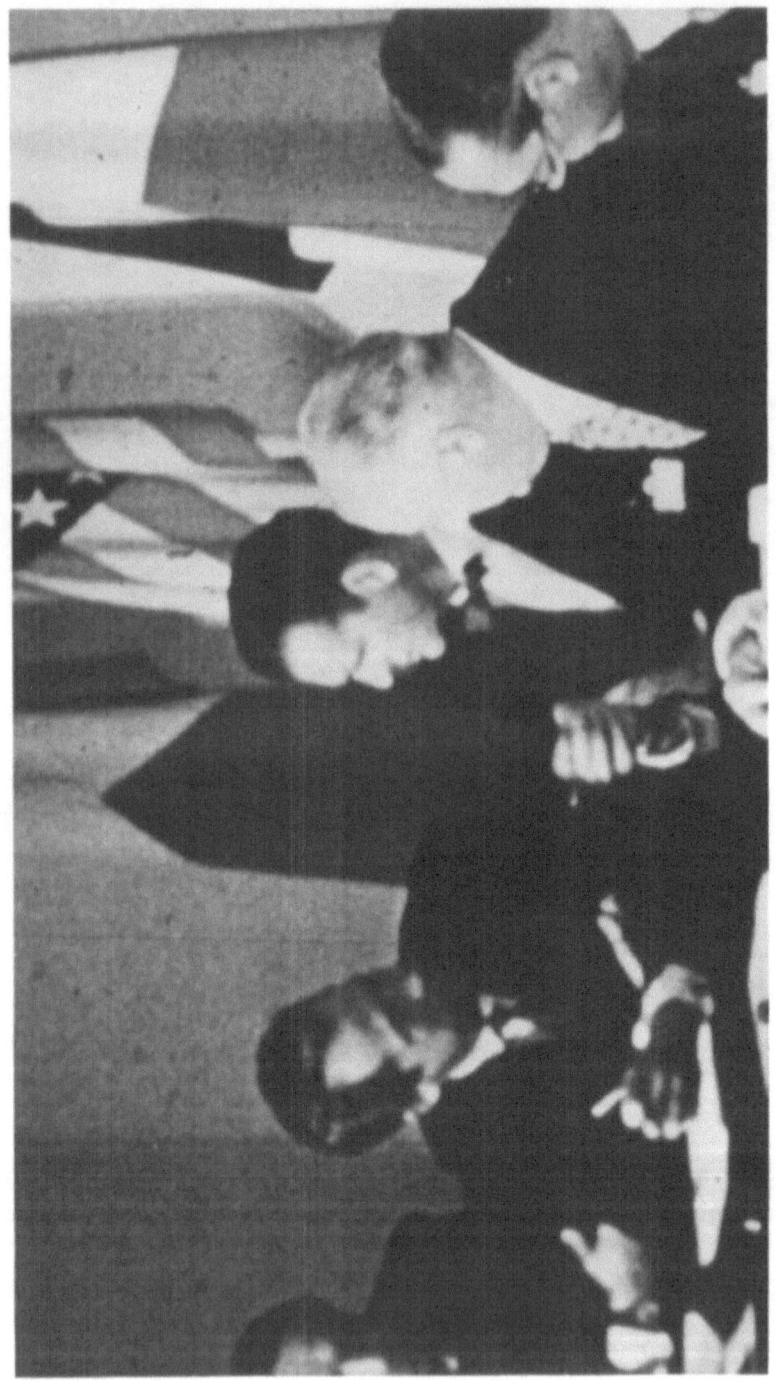

Fig. 3. In 1958, Brom, Senning, Swan and Brock (from left to right) were discussing early open-heart techniques at the European Congress of Cardiology at Brussels with Heim de Balsac as chairman (between Swan and Brock).

Unesco Symposium in Paris in 1961, the entire meeting was devoted to discussion of the use of the heart–lung machine *as a method for the induction of deep hypothermia,* with the idea of turning the machine off for long periods during the operation. Indeed, today deep hypothermia remains the choice of many cardiac surgeons, particularly in Japan, for the correction of complicated congenital malformations in infants, using 60 minutes of circulatory occlusion at 20 °C. And today also, as an integral part of various techniques of cardioplegia to preserve the myocardium during bypass with aortic clamping, general and topical hypothermia remain the fundamental keystone of all techniques. But I am getting ahead of my part of this story.

Mr. Chairman, in 1958, some of the pioneers of open-heart surgery participated in a symposium during the Third World Congress of Cardiology held in Brussels. In Figure 3, one can see a group of five of them seated at the table, and I was apparently losing an argument against overwhelming odds.

By the end of the 1950s, open-heart surgery was a *fait accompli.* In conclusion of this introductory exposition of the history of this rapidly flowering branch of surgery, let me leave you with the memory of how two prominent young pioneers looked at that meeting 21 years ago: our Chairman this morning, Professor Gerry Brom: and our next speaker, Professor Åke Senning.

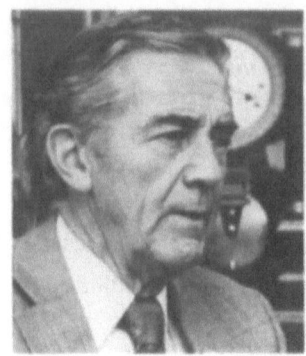

WILLIAM G. BIGELOW

William G. Bigelow is senior cardiac surgeon at the Toronto General Hospital. His group has had considerable long-term success with many mammary-artery implants for myocardial revascularization.

An experiment — cardiac surgery with hypothermia (movie)

Following Dr. Swan's paper, Dr. W.G. Bigelow introduced and showed a four-minute movie, made 28 years ago, for its historical interest. His research in hypothermia started in 1947. Initially it was demonstrated that, contrary to accepted beliefs, the oxygen consumption of an animal was lowered with a fall in body temperature, provided all muscle tremor was eliminated.

In 1950, the use of hypothermia as a means of performing intracardiac surgery was published with evidence that there would be real limitations to safe cooling. A body temperature below 24°–30°C was not safe. As a result, the research continued in two directions: (a) perfecting current techniques to ensure early and late survival, and (b) studying profound hypothermia by research into hibernation.

The movie showed: (a) one of 12 monkeys cooled to 20°C body temperature with 20 minutes open cardiotomy and survival in all – before the technique was first applied to humans by Lewis and Swan, (b) the capture of hibernating groundhogs. They could be artificially cooled to 3°C body temperature with open cardiotomy for two hours and no ill effects.

This tolerance to low body temperature appeared to be related to the presence of hibernating glands. A groundhog farm was established and with help from the best chemists available an attempt was made to obtain an extract from the blood or glands of hibernating groundhogs that would enable safe deep hypothermia in humans. This work continued from 1950 to 1962 without success and the hibernating animals still retain their secret.

148

ÅKE SENNING

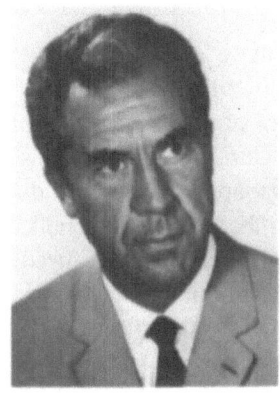

Åke Senning, born in 1915 in Sweden, trained as a general surgeon at various Swedish hospitals and became chief surgeon at the Department of Thoracic Surgery at the Karolinska Institute in Stockholm in 1957. In 1961, he became professor of surgery and chief of the Department of Surgery at the University Hospital of Zürich in Switzerland. He has contributed several innovations in cardiac surgery, pacemaking and, recently, transluminal coronary artery dilatation.

Extracorporeal circulation

Allow me to present to you first a concise history of events leading to the developments of cardiopulmonary bypass and then relate to you my first-hand, personal experience in the years which led to the beginning of open-heart surgery.

The development of extracorporeal circulation (ECC) for open-heart surgery started with organ perfusion by the physiologists. Progress in three different fields finally made modern ECC possible, i.e. control of blood clotting, and construction of pumps and gas exchangers.

In organ perfusions, clotting of the blood was avoided by using defibrinated blood as described by Panum[31] in 1864. Brodie[6] in 1903 found that some unexpected strange reactions, occurring when he used homologous blood, could be avoided with *autologous* blood. Landsteiners[21] discovery in 1910 of the four blood groups made the use of *homologous* blood relatively risk-free.

Many research workers were looking for methods to prevent the coagulation of whole blood. Jacob[18] in 1895 used Hirudin, taken from leeches, and it was injected into the animal shortly before the perfusion started. Today's anticoagulation started with Baskoff's discovery of a hepatophosphatide in 1908, and Howell's phosphatide 'Cephalin' in 1912. Howell's pupil, McLean[30], was assigned to the task of purifying these phosphatides and of the heart phosphatide 'cuorin,' described by Erlandsson. McLean[30] in 1916 found that these phosphatides. especially cuorin, retarded the course of coagulation to a considerable degree: in one typical experiment, from 3 min to more than 6 h. In 1918, Howell and Holt reported a liver extract with a strong anticoagulation activity which they called 'heparin.' Finally, Best in Toronto and Jorpes in Stockholm succeeded in purifying heparin to a degree that it could be used clinically.

Many methods were used to transport the perfusate, and very early the discussion started about continuous or pulsatile flow. Continuous flow was obtained by gravity, pressure bottles, or the ingenious apparatus of Lindberg[24], working with Carrell in 1931, where blood climbed a standing helic with the upper-end rotating horizontally. Frey and Gruber in 1885 used piston pumps to achieve a pulsatile flow. Many different variations of balloon, diaphragm, and bellows pumps were described for experimental and clinical use.

The semipulsating roller-pump commonly used today was introduced in 1924 by the physiologist Beck, in Kiel, for blood transfusions and was then used for perfusion experiments by Issekutz, Bayliss[3], and DeBakey; this pump was also used by Gibbon[15] in his first clinical case in 1953. The greatest problem was to oxygenate the blood and to wash out the CO_2. This problem could be bypassed by using the blood from a donor animal for organ perfusion and returning it to the donor animal, i.e. cross-circulation. Already around 1800, this was used by Bichat for brain circulation in his physiologic studies of '*la vie et la mort.*' In similar experiments, Brown-Sequard[5] could show that the brain was irreparably damaged after less than 5 min of ischemia.

In 1929, Brukhonenko[7] in experimental *total* body cross-perfusion could show that an ischemic heart standstill could be resuscitated after an aortic cross-clamping had been removed. After a series of animal experiments, Varco and Lillehei in April 1954 introduced this method in clinical use for open-heart surgery.

To avoid the problem of blood, foreign material, and gas contact in oxygenators, homologous and heterologous lungs were used to oxygenate blood for organ and whole body perfusions, but finally the work of Campbell showed that heterologous lungs could not be used for clinical purposes, as unexpected pulmonary edemas occurred after 10–180 min.

The first artificial oxygenation seems to have been achieved by bubbling air and, later, oxygen through blood. These methods were used in the oxygenators of Schroeder (1882), Jacobi (1890)[19], and Brodie (1903)[6]; but because of the extensive foaming, bubblers could not be used practically until Clark[8], Gollan[16], and Gupta in 1950 introduced silicone antifoam to de-bubble the blood.

The other possibility of obtaining a gas exchange was to expose the blood as a thin film to oxygen. Frey and Gruber in 1885 for this purpose used rotating drums; Mandel in 1909 [25] let blood float down over glass beads; Hooker[17] used rotating disks, Drinker rotating cylinders in 1915, and Staub in 1929 [34] used vertical screens like Gibbon[13], and Dennis in 1951 [9] used a rotating screen disk in his clinical cases.

Theoretically the best way of gas exchange would be to use a membrane between the gas and the blood, so several types of membranes from cellophane to silicone were tried and in general we all found that the CO_2 exchange was the limiting factor.

Kolff found that the blood was oxygenated in his artificial kidney, and he and Blazer in 1955 described a rotating coil lung. Cloves made a stationary membrane oxygenator in 1955 for clinical use. This was later modified by Pearce and by Lande-Edwards in the LE oxygenator.

In 1948, Crafoord sent me down to the lab, where Björk had done experiments on cerebral perfusion with a rotating disk machine, designed by Anderson and Crafoord. I was assigned the task of enlarging this machine to be used for total perfusion. A time full of disappointment, but at the same time full of fun, started. It seemed to me that rotating disk oxygenators needed too much blood volume in the trough to get a sufficient oxygen capacity. Therefore, in cooperation with engineer Åstradsson from AGA, we changed to rotating screen cylinders. This gave us an oxygenator and automatic pump that enabled us to perform total body perfusion of 35- to 40-kg dogs at normal temperature with a clamped pulmonary artery. To avoid air embolism and to simplify surgery, we induced ventricular fibrillation and found that the heart could be defibrillated even after hours. It seemed to be a perfect method to prevent air embolism.

Now contacts with other countries started. In 1951, I visited Utrecht, where Gerard Brom worked together with Jongbloed, who had made a monstrous machine, oxygenating blood in several parallel rotating plastic helices. Brom had conducted a series of dog experiments, but the results did not make him believe much in the safety and efficiency of the machine, and Jongbloed doubted, of course, the surgical skill involved. In 1951, at the ICVS meeting in Paris, ECC was a main theme and the first experimental successes were reported. At this same meeting, we met Bill Bigelow, who reported on hypothermia as a method to enable prolongated circulatory arrest. He had opened the heart of 12 monkeys during 20 min at 20 °C body temperature and all animals were rescuscitated and survived. Shortly afterward, Juvenelle came to our lab from Canada, bringing enthusiasm for hypothermia with him. With Lind, Wegelius, and myself, the experiments with combination of ECC and hypothermia were started. It was soon clear that the ECC at a body temperature of 20°–27 °C gave a much broader safety margin. When the tube blew, as it often happened, we had time to repair it. A small air embolus did not seem to be so harmful. A lower flow could be kept without seriously weak heart action afterward. The most important fact was that 3- to 4-h total perfusion experiments started to be successful when ECC was combined with hypothermia.

In 1954, together with the engineer Åstradsson, I visited Jack Gibbon in

Philadelphia. Gibbon[15] had done his first successful case – a girl with an ASD – in 1953. We learned that he had tried three more cases without success and therefore stopped this type of surgery. We were allowed to carefully study his machine and we were very happy to learn his views on extracorporeal circulation – at a dinner in his home. He told us to go to Minneapolis to Wangensteen's clinic where Clarence Dennis had done two clinical cases with his own lung machine. Dennis's first case, in December 1951, was considered to be an ASD. When the heart was opened, none of the surgeons understood the malformation: It was a total AV canal. No correction could be done and the patient died.

The next patient operated on, in January 1952, had an ASD. This was successfully closed, but in the enthusiasm finishing the ECC the pump was not carefully controlled and, at the end, pumped the oxygenator trough empty and the patient full of air. No more clinical cases were made with this machine.

Wangensteen sent me down to the lab to see what he thought to be very promising experiments on controlled low cross-circulation. I met Walt Lillehei, who performed the experiments. Unfortunately, no dogs were available. I saw only some sigma motor pumps and tubings, but – after a couple of dry Martini's, a good dinner, and some whisky at 4 o'clock in the morning – I think I had learned enough of cross-circulation and had decided not to try it.

Lillehei and Varco thought differently and two months later, in April 1954, they started a series of 45 infant operations in which one of the parents was the donor – 'a better heart lung machine cannot be found' – according to Lillehei. Lillehei and Varco pioneered with the first corrections of VSDs, Fallot's tetralogy, etc.

When they reported to the New York Academy in 1955 on their correction of Fallot's tetralogy with four of seven patients surviving the operation, our grand lady today, Dr. Taussig, was not very happy and said – as far as I remember – 'I am unhappy that they had any survivals at all, because now others will try' – and they did.

There was an enormous amount of experimental work done in the USA to develop the heart–lung machine – at the same time also in several centers in Europe, e.g. in London: in Hammersmith by Cleland, Melrose[26], and Bental; and in Guy's Hospital by Brock's team; and in Paris, Turin, and Stockholm.

In 1951, Dogliotti[10] in Turin had made a partial bypass with a bubbler when operating a tracheal tumor. At Hammersmith in London, Cleland in December 1953, using Melrose's machine, explored a mitral valve in total bypass but could not do anything to correct the valvular insufficiency. The patient survived the exploration. Three more operations were performed, but all of the patients died.

In Stockholm, our lab work was so far advanced that Crafoord in July 1954 decided to operate on a 42-year-old woman with a severe left heart insufficiency and systemic artery emboli caused by a pseudomyxoma in the left auricle. The patient was placed on the operating table on a plastic sheet and planks were placed around the patient to form a trough which was filled with ice water. She was now surface-cooled to 26 °C. The water and the planks were removed and the operation performed with ventricular fibrillation induced for cardiac standstill. During this period, the pseudomyxoma in the left auricle was removed. This patient is still living and free from symptoms.

We started to get the first monitoring instruments. Elema had built an oscilloscope for me, with 17 vacuum tubes, but an intensive care unit did not exist. The patient was left – after rewarming – on the operating table till next morning. I was resting on a stretcher next to her.

During 1955, several clinics in the USA as well as in Europe started open-heart surgery and an increasing number of successes were reported. As the National Heart Institute had given enormous support to the research on heart–lung machines, the national Advisory Heart Council suggested a conference to be held to discuss the developments in this field, and this conference was realized in Edgewaters Beach Hotel in September 1957. About 220 research workers in this field from the USA, Canada, and Europe were invited. During the meeting, practically all aspects of the technique of extracorporeal circulation were discussed – during the day in the lecture room and during the night (perhaps more intensively) in various bars and nightclubs.

The machines reported were not so sophisticated as today, but in principle very little has changed since then. The bubblers had not yet shown their superiority to the film or membrane oxygenators, and the discussion on continuous or pulsatile flow is still not finished. Flow rates, the problem of embolization, cardioplegia with potassium citrate (Melrose) or acetylcholin (Lam) were discussed, and the final decisions seem all correct even today.

When we look back on the last two decades, we find that nothing really new has happened to the ECC. The machines are refined and our surgical technique has become routine; even if it has not yet reached perfection, it is good enough to enable us to treat infants of a few weeks and old people of 70 years or more of age, and to diminish the mortality from about 35% to 40% for VSD, and Fallot's tetralogy corrections to about 1%, 3%, 4% in different cardiac malformations.

The real progress has taken place in the postoperative care in the intensive care unit with a huge amount of instruments monitoring all aspects of hemodynamic, respiratory, and metabolic changes.

To assist a failing heart not responding enough on inotropic drugs, Moulopoulos et al. in 1961 [29] introduced the intraaortic balloon pumping experimentally. Since Kantrowitz's trial with infarcted patients, it has gained widespread use in most countries in postoperative left heart failure. We have learned to correct some of the mistakes we did during surgery, e.g. damage to the His bundle when closing defects. The introduction of pacemakers not only decreased surgical mortality but it also found a wide use in cardiology.

The pump assist as a left and, if necessary, a right heart bypass to temporarily support a failling heart, has in some cases been beneficial, but its deleterious effect on blood and especially on the coagulation system still makes its use justified in only a limited number of cases.

The cardiorespiratory-supporting machines and, above all, the oxygen–blood interphase have to be perfected so that they can be used for days and weeks.

REFERENCES

1. Aguilar MJ, Gerbode F, Hill JD (1971) Neuropathologic complications of cardiac surgery. J Thorac Cardiovasc Surg 61:676
2. Garrott AJ (1958) Extracorporeal circulation. Springfield IL: Charles C Thomas
3. Bayliss LE, Fee AR, Ogden E (1928) A method of oxygenating blood. J Physiol 66:443
4. Bainbridge FA, Evans CL (1914) The heart, lung, kidney preparation. J Physiol 48:278
5. Brown-Séquard E (1858) Recherches expérimentales sur les propriétés physiologiques et les usages du sang rouge et du sang noir et leurs principaux éléments gazeux, L'oxygène et l'acide carbonique. J Physiol Homme (Paris) 1:95
6. Brodie TG (1903) The perfusion of surviving organs. J Physiol 29:266
7. Brukhonenko S (1929) Circulation artificielle du sang dans l'organisme entier d'un chien avec cœur exclu. J Physiol Pathol Gen 27:257
8. Clark LC Jr, Gollan G, Gupta V (1950) The oxygenation of blood by gas dispersion. Science 111:85
9. Dennis C, Spreng DS, et al. (1955) Development of a pump oxygenator to replace the heart and lungs: apparatus applicable to human patients and application in one case. Ann Surg 134:709
10. Dogliotti AM, et al. (1961) Extracorporeal circulation in deep hypothermia: an experimental study. J Int Coll Surg 35:302
11. Embley EH, Martin MB (1905) The action of anaesthetic quantities of chloroform upon the blood vessels of the bowel and kidney with an account of an artificial circulation apparatus. J Physiol 32:147
12. Fleisch A (1935) Ein automatisch regulierender Durchblutungsapparat mit fortlaufender Registrierung der Durchblutungsgeschwindigkeit. Handbuch biol Arbeitsmethoden, München, Teil 8, p 1007
13. Gibbon JH (1938) An oxygenator with a large surface volume ratio. J Lab Clin Med 24:1192
14. Gibbon JH (1939) The maintenance of life during experimental occlusion of the pulmonary artery followed by survival. Surg Gynecol Obstet 69:602
15. Gibbon JH (1954) Application of a mechanical heart and lung apparatus to cardiac surgery. Minn Med 37:171
16. Gollan F (1959) Physiology of cardiac surgery. Springfield IL: Charles C Thomas
17. Hooker DR (1915) The perfusion of the mammalian medulla – the effect of calcium and potassium on the respiratory and cardiac centers. Am J Physiol 38:200

18. Jacobj C (1895) Ein Beitrag zur Technik der künstlichen Durchblutung überlebender Organe. Arch Exp Pathol 36:330
19. Jacobj D (1890) Apparat zur Durchblutung isolierter überlebender Organe. Arch Exp Pathol 26:388
20. Kingsbury FB (1916) Perfusion pump. J Biol Chem 28:166
21. Landsteiner K (1901) Über Agglutinationserscheinungen normalen menschlichen Blutes. Wien Klin Wochenschr 14:1132
22. Langendorff O (1897) Untersuchungen am überlebenden Säugetierherzen. II. Abhandlung. Arch Ges Physiol 66:355
23. Leusner B (1971) Grundversuche in der Entwicklung der Maschine. Inaug Diss Med Fak Köln, 13 Feb
24. Lindbergh CA (1935) An apparatus for the culture of whole organs. J Exp Med 62:409
25. Mandel F (1908) Ein neuer Apparat zur Durchblutung überlebender Organe. Z Biol Tech Meth 1:44
26. Melrose D (1955) Elective cardiac arrest. Lancet, 21 July
27. Meneely GR, Ferguson JL (1961) Pulmonary evaluation and risk in patients' preparation for anaesthesia and surgery. JAMA 175:122
28. Miller WF Wu N, Johnson RL (1956) Convenient method of evaluating pulmonary ventilatory function with a single breath test. Anaesthesiology 17:480
29. Mounopoulos Sp, Topaz St, et al. (1962) Diastolic balloon pumping with carbon dioxide in the aorta. A mechanical assistance to the failing circulation. Am Heart J 63:669
30. McLean (1916) Am J Physiol 41:250
31. Panum PL (1864) Experimentelle Untersuchungen über die Transfusion, Transplantation oder Substitution des Blutes in theoretischer und praktischer Beziehung. Virchows Arch Pathol Anat 240 (Arch Anat Physiol)
32. Rosenberger H (1930) An electromagnetic pump. Science 71:463
33. Senning Å (1962) Herzchirurgie – gestern, heute und morgen. Vortrag
34. Staub H (1929) Methode zur fortlaufenden Bestimmung des Gaswechsels isoliert durchströmter Organe im geschlossenen System. Arch Exp Pathol Pharmakol 162:420
35. Wiggers CJ (1960) Some significant advances in cardiac physiology during the nineteenth century. Bull Hist Med 34:1

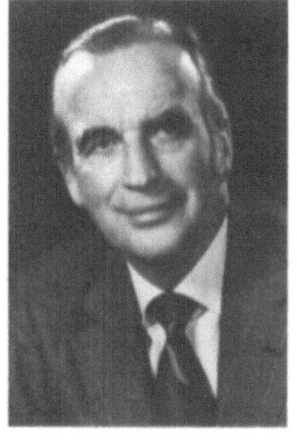

DONALD B. EFFLER

Donald B. Effler, born 1915, was chief of the Department of Thoracic and Cardiovascular Surgery at the Cleveland Clinic Foundation from 1949 till 1975. Following the anatomical documentation of coronary artery disease by selective catheterization, pioneered by Dr. Mason Sones at the same institution, Dr. Effler and his team started saphenous vein graft techniques in 1967 for revascularization of the heart. He has greatly contributed to the development and safety of coronary artery surgery.

Surgery of ischemic heart disease

Modern revascularization surgery was introduced by selective coronary arteriography (Sones' technique) in 1959. The earliest efforts to introduce a new source of saturated blood to ischemic myocardium included the Vineberg Internal Mammary Implant Procedure, coronary endarterectomy, and coronary artery patch grafts. Of these methods, the internal mammary implant procedure had the broadest application and many patients did benefit by this indirect approach to direct revascularization.

The saphenous vein graft techniques and internal mammary artery–coronary artery grafts received clinical application in 1967, and these direct approaches to revascularization are used widely in many parts of the world today. The selection of patients for revascularization surgery and the final evaluation of the surgical result depend upon cine-coronary arteriogram and ventriculography.

As would be expected, a variety of methods for accomplishing the same mission have evolved. Surgeons have rediscovered so-called myocardial preservation techniques that include hypothermia, coronary artery perfusion, chemical cardioplegia, and intraaortic balloon assist. Cardiologists and cardiovascular surgeons alike refer to revascularization as 'complete or incomplete – adequate or inadequate.' The exact meaning of these descriptive terms varies widely, but the inescapable fact remains that revascularization surgery must relieve a myocardial perfusion deficit if the optimal result is to be obtained. More than 12 years have elapsed since the introduction of the bypass graft techniques that utilize veins or mammary arteries; truth and fallacy have emerged, but the fact remains that the surgical treatment of ischemic heart disease will relieve pain, prevent infarction, and prolong life.

157

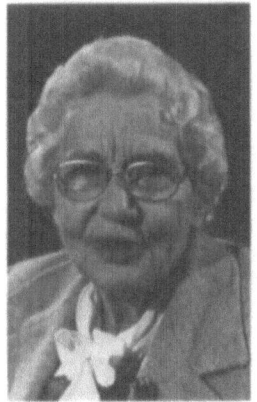

Helen B. Taussig, born in 1898, was in charge of the pediatric cardiac clinic at Johns Hopkins School of Medicine from 1930 till 1963 and professor of pediatrics at the institution from 1959 till 1963. In 1947, she wrote 'Congenital malformations of the heart', a classic description of congenital heart disease, its hemodynamics, and its clinical symptoms and signs, at the start of its surgical management. Together with the surgeon Dr. Alfred Blalock, she worked on the development of the Blalock–Taussig systemic-pulmonary shunt operation and did a long follow-up on its results. Today she is still active in the prevention of congenital malformations, which started with the thalidomide drama in 1962. Also, she is actively supporting women's rights, especially for abortion, and the right to die with dignity.

Personal memories of surgery of tetralogy

Dr. Edwards A. Park, Pediatrician in Chief of the Johns Hopkins School of Medicine, and Chief of the Harriet Lane Home for Invalid Children (Fig. 1), put me in charge of his new pediatric cardiac clinic in 1930. Although the clinic was established primarily for children with acute rheumatic fever and rheumatic heart disease, all types of cardiac complications were referred to the clinic, including patients with congenital malformations of the heart. The little cyanotic babies were regularly referred, as nothing could be done for them.

I examined them as carefully as I did patients with acquired heart disease. Gradually I came to realize that the cyanotic infants with pulmonary atresia died as the ductus closed, and those with severe pulmonary stenosis became markedly worse. This set me thinking on how to keep the ductus open. In 1939, when Gross and Hubbard showed it was surgically possible to ligate a ductus, I immediately thought that it must be possible for a surgeon to build a ductus. Indeed, I went to Boston and asked Dr. Gross whether he could build a ductus. He replied that he had built many, but he was not at all interested in my idea. It was a happy day for me when Dr. Blalock came to Baltimore. He had successfully ligated the ductus arteriosus in three patients (Fig. 2).

Dr. Park immediately tried to interest Dr. Blalock in developing an operation for coarctation of the aorta. I took courage and selected a patient with a patent ductus arteriosus for operation. At the end of the operation, I said to Dr. Blalock, 'I stand in awe and admiration of your surgical skill, but the truly great day will come when you build a ductus for a child dying of anoxemia and not when you ligate a ductus for a child who has a little too

159

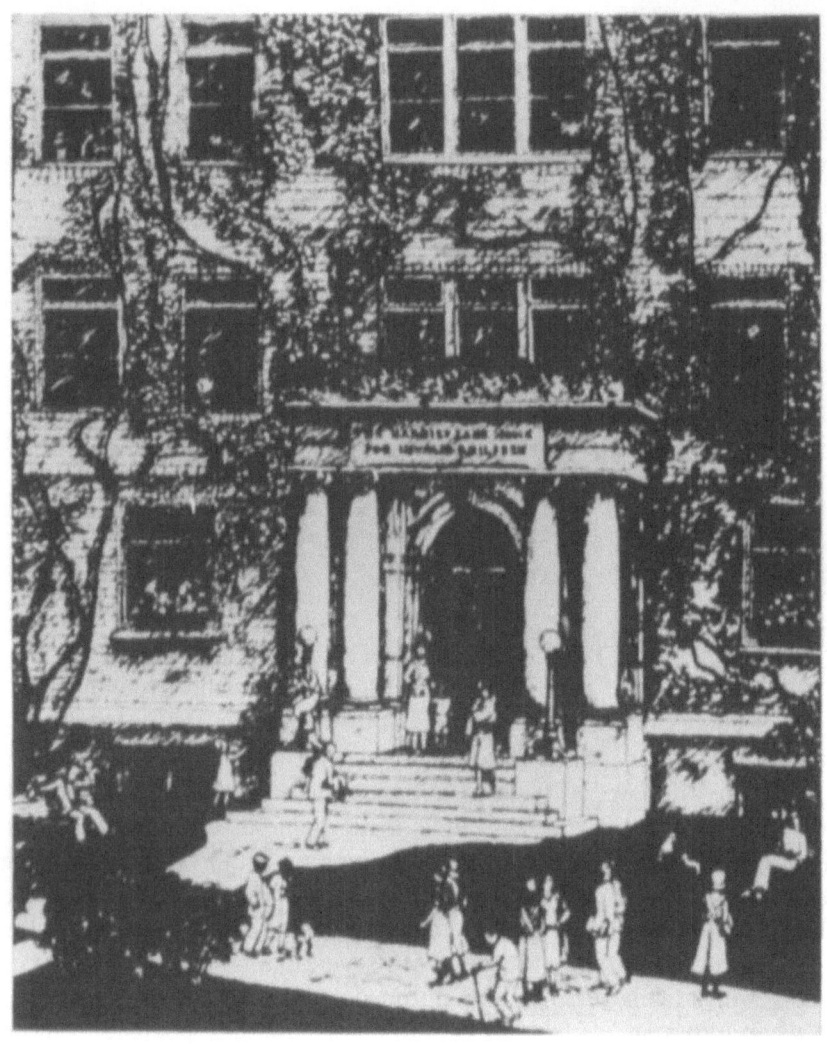

Fig. 1. Harriet Lane Home for Invalid Children.

much blood going to his lungs.' Dr. Blalock replied, 'When that day comes, this will seem like child's play.' Two years later, he did his first anastomosis!

During the intervening two years, Dr. Blalock took the problem to his laboratory as he had done with Dr. Park's suggestion of devising an operation for coarction of the aorta. Dr. Blalock thought that if one could cross-clamp the aorta in a normal dog and do an end-to-end anastomosis on the aorta, one could safely cross-clamp the aorta if the person had a coarctation of the aorta with extensive collateral circulation. It so happened that the first six dogs developed paralysis of the lower extremities. When Dr. Blalock reported his difficulty at a pediatric X-ray conference, Dr. Park pointed out that the

160

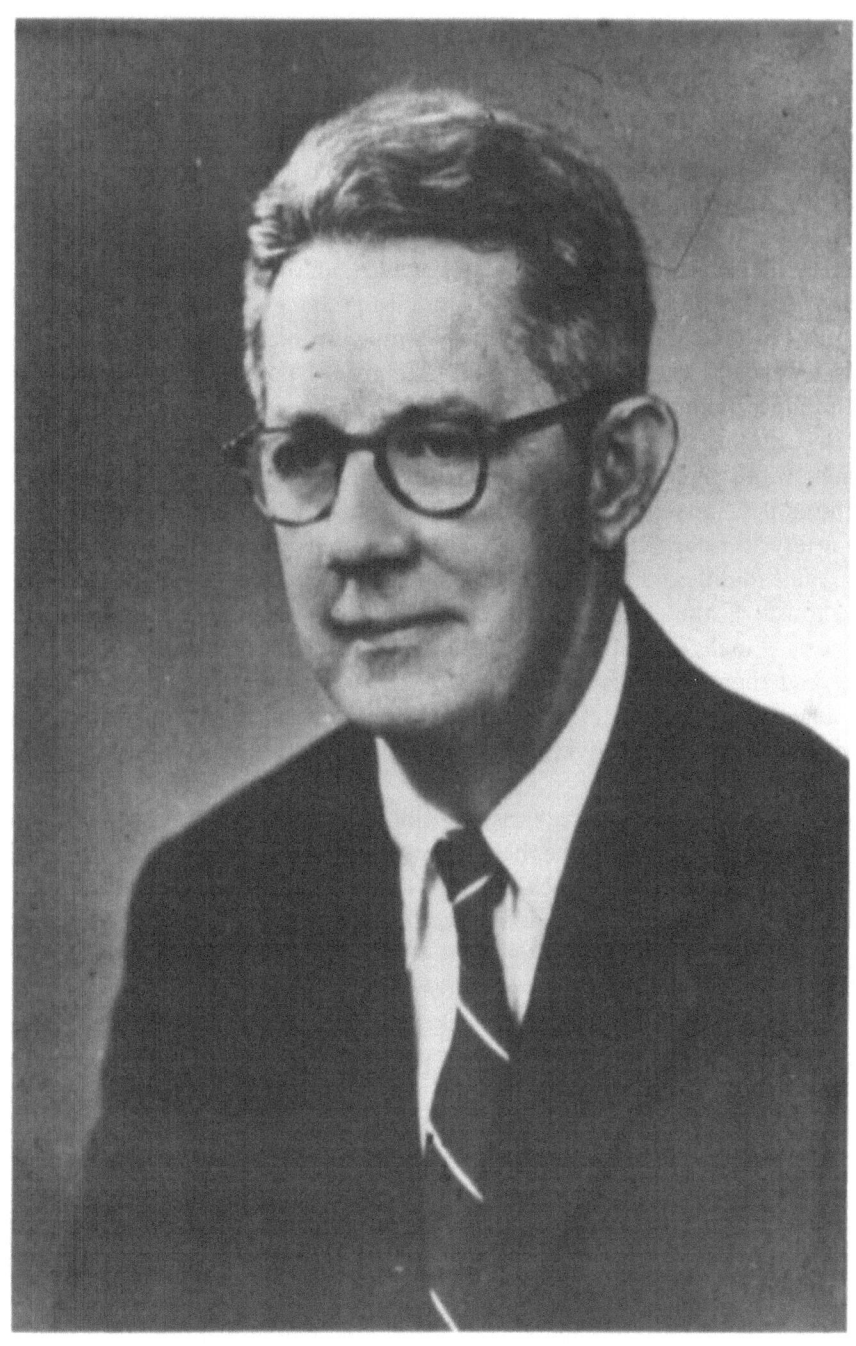

Fig. 2. Dr. Alfred Blalock.

carotid artery was a long straight vessel and there were four arteries to the brain and ample collateral circulation. Then he asked Dr. Blalock whether he could not bring down the left carotid artery and anastomose it to the aorta below the coarctation. I immediately said, 'Could you not anastomose the subclavian artery to the pulmonary artery? That is all I want.' Dr. Blalock replied by inviting me to his laboratory.

There I met Vivian Thomas – that remarkable black technician whom Dr. Blalock had trained and who later received an honorary degree from the Johns Hopkins University. He was trying to produce pulmonary stenosis. The ligatures around the pulmonary artery simply worked their way through the vessel wall and caused no pulmonary stenosis. I pointed out that even if it did produce pulmonary stenosis in a normal heart, it would not cause cyanosis. I suggested that he put the right pulmonary artery into the left auricle, which would direct venous blood to the left side of the heart. Then when cyanosis developed, he could put the left subclavian artery into the pulmonary artery to relieve the cyanosis. Vivian Thomas did the first step the next day, but the dog did not develop cyanosis. Next he combined a partial lobectomy of the right lung with the anastomosis, but that too gave no cyanosis. Finally Vivian Thomas removed all but the upper lobe of the right lung and thereby got some cyanosis. After experiments on nearly 200 dogs, Dr. Blalock said to me, 'The experiments are suggestive but not very conclusive. But if you are convinced the operation will work, I am convinced I know how to do it.'

At that time there was a little 13-month-old cyanotic baby on the ward who weighed but 10 lbs. and had been living in an oxygen tent for several months. We asked Dr. Blalock whether he would consider operating on such a poor risk. He replied, 'That is the sort of patient on whom one should try a new operation.' The parents realized that some sort of operation was the infant's only hope and readily gave consent.

On November 29, 1944, Dr. Blalock performed his first 'blue baby' operation. He was disappointed at the small size of the subclavian artery: it was no bigger than a matchstick. He felt no thrill, but did think blood was going through it to the lungs. The baby had a stormy postoperative course, but survived.

In January 1945, we discussed which tests might measure the results (we hoped improvements) of the operations. Early in February, Dr. Blalock performed his second operation. The patient was an 11-year-old deeply cyanotic girl with 10 million red blood cells who was losing consciousness several times a day for half an hour at a time. She had a right aortic arch. Dr. Blalock decided to operate on the left as he had done before. He reached high up into the apex of the chest in an effort to get a large vessel. He brought down the innominate artery and anastomosed it to the pulmonary artery. On

162

release of the clamps, he felt a beautiful thrill but we saw no appreciable change in color. It was not till three weeks later, when she walked down the corridor to meet her father, that we appreciated how great her improvement was.

It was not until the third operation that we saw a dramatic change in color. The patient was a six-year-old, miserably unhappy, deeply cyanotic boy who could no longer walk. Obviously he needed a large vessel: so Dr. Blalock operated on the right chest, as the boy had a normal left aortic arch. Dr. Blalock again used the innominate artery. On release of the clamps, blood welled up into the chest. Quickly Dr. Blalock located the bleeding point. He sewed it up and, knowing the boy had 10 million red blood cells, he poured in plasma. When he next released the clamps, he said, 'I feel a beautiful thrill' and almost simultaneously the anesthesiologist called out, 'He is a *lovely* color now.' I walked to the head of the table and saw the child with bright pink cheeks and cherry red lips! The child woke up in the operating room and asked to get up. We knew we had won.

Dr. Blalock did a few more innominate anastomosis, and then when he saw a good-sized subclavian artery, he used it and got a good result. The second time he used the subclavian branch of the innominate artery, we realized it made a smoother anastomosis than was possible with the subclavian artery which arose from the aorta. Thereafter, the standard operation for an infant or child was to operate on the opposite side to the aortic arch and anastomose the subclavian branch of the innominate artery to the side of the left or right main pulmonary artery.

By now you are all familiar with the long-term results.

To Dr. Blalock's great credit, 10% of the patients whom he operated upon between 1945 and 1951, and who survived the operation, were well and living active lives 20–28 years after his/her first and only cardiac surgery.

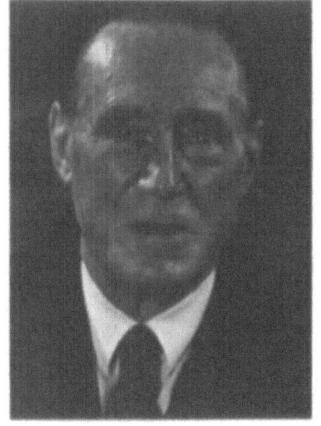

LORD BROCK†

Lord Brock, born in 1903, was thoracic surgeon both at Guy's and the Brompton Hospital in London from 1936 till 1968. Shortly after the war, he was the first to attack valvular obstruction in the heart, and he performed valvotomy for pulmonary stenosis in 1948, followed by infundibular resection in Fallot's tetralogy. Against much scepsis, he successfully did the first mitral commissurotomies in that same year, opening the road to valvular heart surgery by the closed approach. Lord Brock died ten months after the Einthoven meeting.

Personal memories of the early days of cardiac valve surgery

The basic functions of surgery are the control of haemorrhage, the care of wounds, the mending of broken bones and the relief of an obstruction to a hollow viscus or duct. It is well known that this latter is fundamental in the case of the urinary tract, the gallbladder and bile duct system, but for a long time it was ignored in the case of the cardiovascular system. It was rejected or denied for perhaps two reasons. Firstly it was thought to be impractical and secondly many were against it on principle.

Moreover it was thought that valve obstruction did not primarily matter but it was the myocardium that mattered, indeed the surgeon who thought otherwise was an ignorant, even dangerous individual. The approach to cardiology was essentially medical. For centuries, cardiology had been, as it were, protected against surgery. Heart disease was essentially a medical condition and no surgeon should be encouraged to look upon it as in his province.

I was personally greatly inspired by the success of Henry Souttar in 1925 in demonstrating that it was possible to operate on the mitral valve. This very success saw the arrest of all progress in valve surgery. Souttar was not working closely with his cardiological colleagues and at his hospital there was a strong medical, almost anti-surgical, approach. His patient came to him direct from a general practitioner and in fact did not have mitral stenosis. It is evident from his account of the operation that she had dominant severe mitral regurgitation and died from this some five years later. No further patient was sent to him nor was likely to be by his cardiological colleagues at Sir James Mackenzie's old hospital. Although misguided, Souttar had sown the seed and this encouraged others, e.g. Evarts Graham and especially the Boston group headed by Cutler and Levine. Again no real success was achieved and this further strengthened the case against surgery; the time was not yet favourable. I well remember that when I approached one cardiologist, incidentally a personal friend, I received an answer that surely I knew that it had been conclusively shown that surgery had no place in the treatment of mitral stenosis and that I ought to be fully aware of this. I remembered this comment a year or two later when the floodgates were open and we were deluged with the demands, essentially from patients, for mitral valvotomy.

But I must leave mitral valvotomy for the time being and return to other aspects of valve surgery. The whole world was impressed with the epoch-making work of Blalock and Taussig, who not only showed that great success

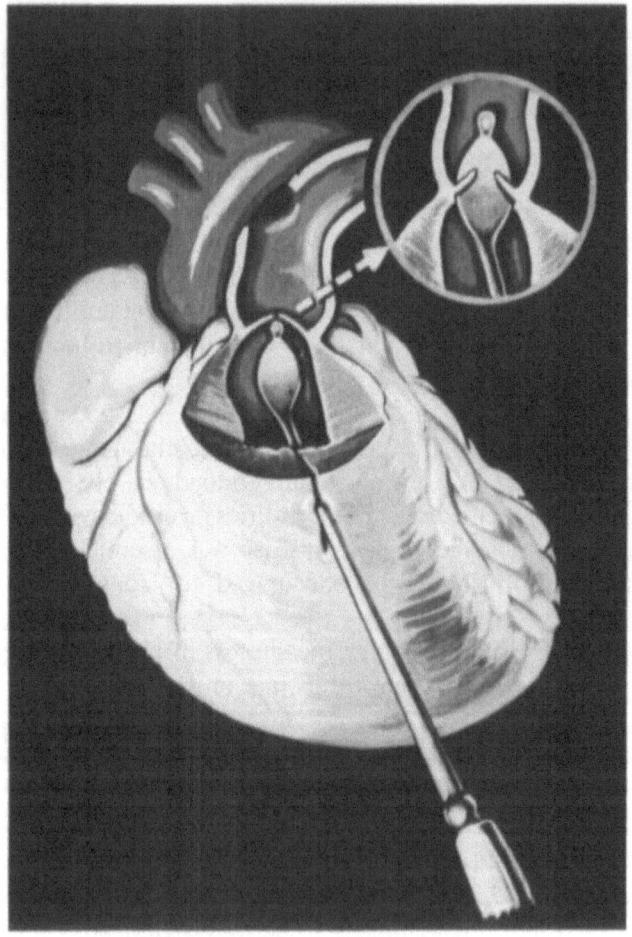

Fig. 1. Diagram to show closed pulmonary valvotomy.

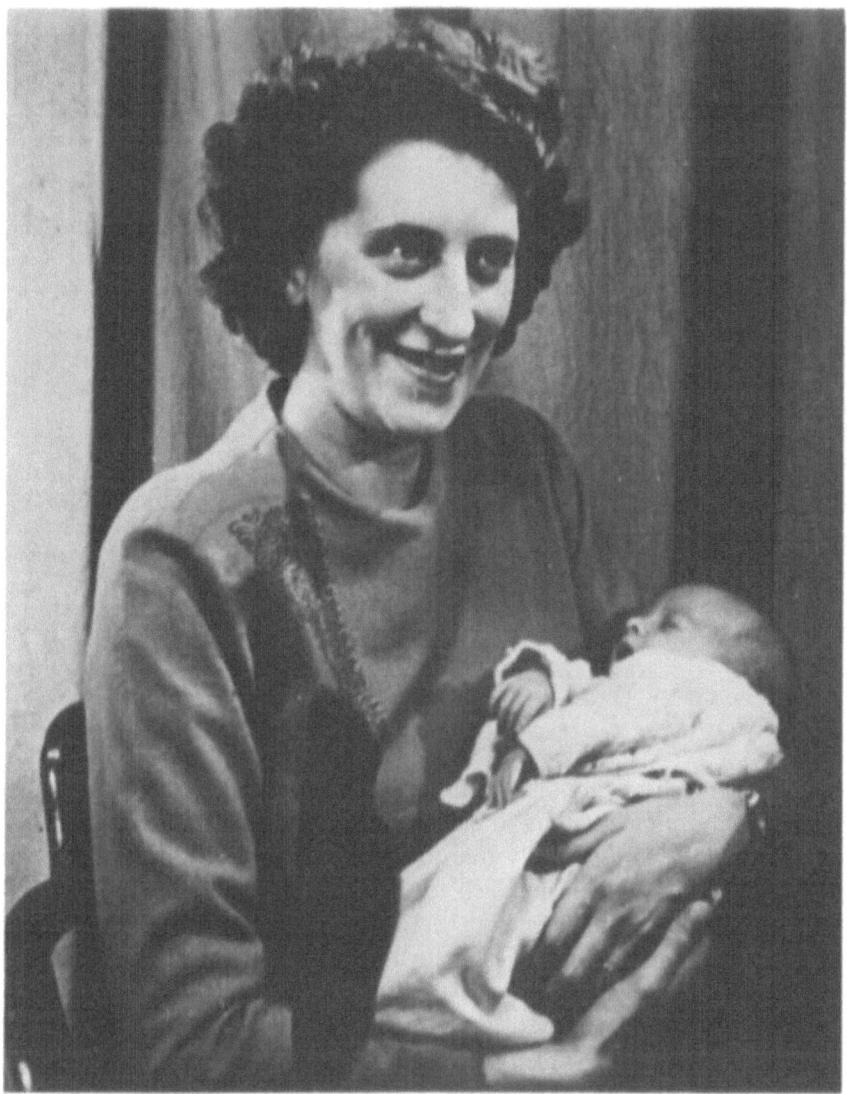

Fig. 2. Patient 12 months after operation.

could be achieved with a previously hopeless condition, the blue baby, but also that it could be done by an indirect operation and one not directly on the heart itself. The obstruction could be by-passed or short-circuited by an arterial anastomosis around it. Blalock at that time was doing experimental research on pulmonary hypertension by joining a systemic artery to the pulmonary artery, and Dr. Helen Taussig had the brilliant idea that cyanosis might be relieved by bringing more blood to the lungs by an anastomosis of the Blalock type. Success was immediate and so outstanding that it altered

167

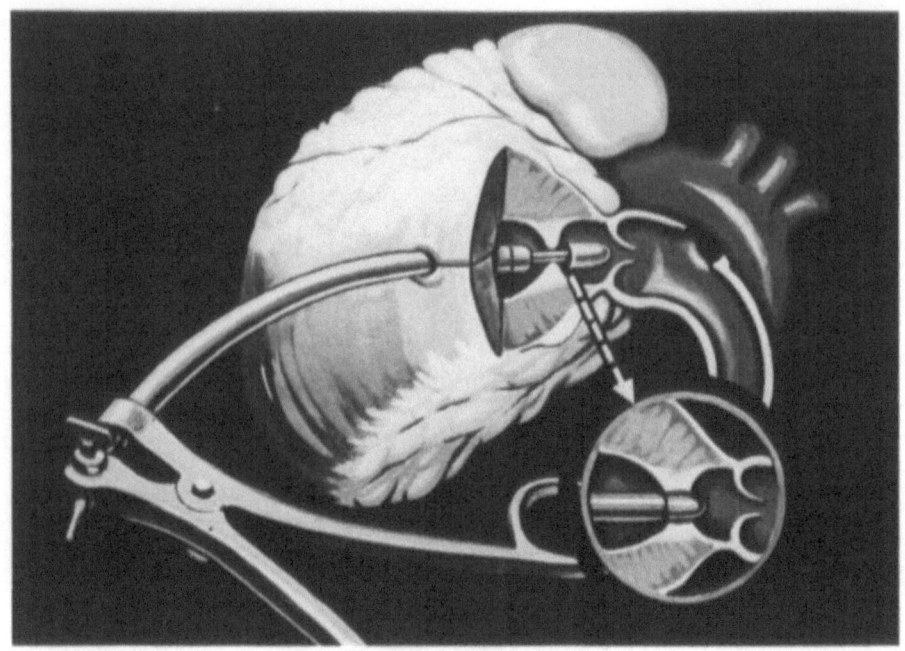

Fig. 3. Method of closed infundibular resection.

the whole approach to cardiology and now offered a hope of cure. Although I was profoundly impressed by their results, I still had some reservations. Fallot's tetralogy was essentially due to an obstruction within the heart itself and I felt that the sounder approach to the problem should be direct relief of the stenosis, which would benefit the heart by taking away the obstruction rather than by adding another lesion to the burden the heart was carrying.

This was rendered more difficult for me because in 1947 Alfred Blalock came to Guy's Hospital as visiting surgeon and did ten operations for cyanotic heart disease, all of which were completely and brilliantly successful. A great achievement. After his return home, I was deluged with cases for operation, but I continued to have doubts about the soundness of the conception of indirect surgery as opposed to a direct attack upon the stenosis. I looked for possible favourable cases and eventually in 1948 I was able to report three cases in which I had been successful in doing a pulmonary valvotomy, a direct relief of the obstruction (Fig. 1). This was not too enthusiastically received by my colleagues; indeed one cardiologist said that I had no right to take such a risk when an operation of proven worth was already in existence! I lost touch with one of these three patients when she went to Canada, but the other two I followed for over 20 years; one had two healthy children (Fig. 2).

168

The year 1948 was an *annus mirabilis* for me and, in addition to doing pulmonary valvotomy for Fallot's tetralogy, I also did my first closed infundibular resection (Fig. 3), the patient is still alive and well 30 years later, and also my first mitral valvotomy to which I shall return later. In addition I was also successful in performing my first pulmonary valvotomy for cyanotic heart disease. I feel that perhaps this was my greatest success in this disease and I still feel so.

In 1949, it fell to me to go to the Johns Hopkins Hospital as visiting professor of surgery and I renewed my happy contact with Alfred Blalock and Helen Taussig. The first patient I was asked to operate on was a boy of 14 who had had a Blalock's operation a year earlier. His cyanosis had disappeared, but he was in right-sided heart failure and Dr. Taussig realised that instead of Fallot's tetralogy he had pulmonary valve stenosis with an intact ventricular septum and an atrial communication. The ventricle could not support the extra strain of the anastomosis. The pulmonary valvotomy went well, but instead of being content with this, I proceeded to do what I should have left for another day, namely to undo the subclavian–pulmonary anastomosis. I

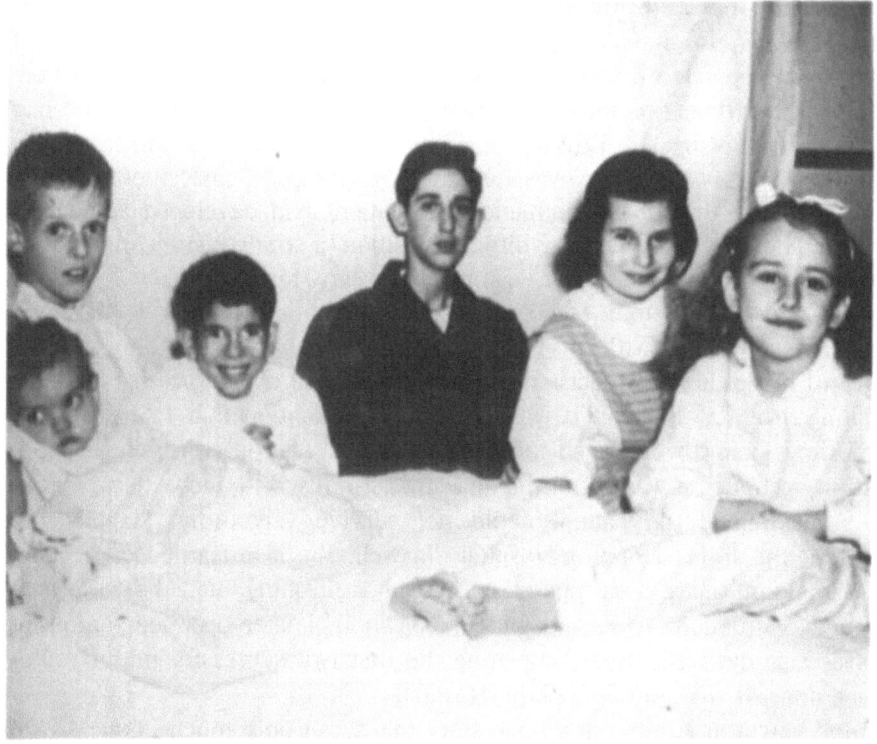

Fig. 4. A group of six patients all of whom had had pulmonary valvotomy in the three preceding weeks.

was well into this procedure when the patient's heart stopped and I failed to revive it. Dr. Taussig with her great wisdom and kindness said to me that she fully approved of what I had done and would like me to operate on more of her patients.

Thus, the very next day, I did a pulmonary valvotomy on another child; this time with complete success and I am able to show you this photograph of six patients who had been blue and on whom I did a successful pulmonary valvotomy (Fig. 4). They include a baby aged 14 months, who was also in right-sided failure, having had a Potts' operation. On this occasion I was tempted, and after the valvotomy I closed the Potts' anastomosis without event. All these patients remain well up to date, 30 years after. The baby has, in fact, distinguished himself by going to prison.

I have had many excellent and long-lasting results from infundibular resection and at one time I had thought this would be all that was necessary. Now, as a result of a fuller experience, I realise that total correction should always be aimed at, that is in addition to closure of the septal defect, a thorough clearance of the obstruction in the outflow tract, both muscular and valvar, is needed.

I must now revert to mitral stenosis and valvotomy. Before I went to the Johns Hopkins Hospital, I had done five successful mitral valvotomies and I was asked to operate on some patients at the Johns Hopkins Hospital, where none had been done previously. My first patient was a man aged 31 who had been looked after by Dr. Taussig for many years. I was faced with a terrible decision which at that time was quite new to me. The anaesthetist sent a message to say that during induction the patient had developed acute pulmonary oedema. I was in a very difficult position, a stranger surgeon about to do a new type of operation at a leading American Hospital where it had not only not been done before, but there was much scepticism about it. Moreover I had already failed with my first case of pulmonary valvotomy. Thank Heaven I made the right decision to proceed with the operation; in this I was encouraged by Dr. Blalock. It was, of course, a situation that I was to meet many times before we learned to guard against it. The only occasion I had a death in such a case was when the anaesthetist refused to allow me to go on, as he maintained the patient could not survive valvotomy. Happily my patient at the Johns Hopkins Hospital did well. We also learned once again the paramount place that operation has in controlling an otherwise fatal obstructive situation. A second patient on whom I later operated for mitral stenosis also did well, thus completing the first two successful mitral valvotomies done at the Johns Hopkins Hospital.

Mitral valvotomy presents a huge story that I can only touch upon. As we all know, when the floodgates were opened we were faced with a torrent of patients who demanded operation, even though they often received little medical encouragement. Put briefly, the initial operative approach to the problem was all wrong and in fact ignored the anatomical features of the stenosed valve state. To the early surgeons, a small hole was just a hole and should be enlarged.

Hence Cutler and his associates and also Evarts Graham attempted to use a cardioscope that could be introduced into the heart and then used to punch out a piece of the rim of the valve orifice or cut into it. Graham did have the extra idea of introducing his instrument through the atrial appendage and not through the ventricle.

My study of the mitral valve showed me that the stenosis was the result of fusion of the two cusps antermedially and posterolaterally in such a way that demanded an oblique approach to separate them; that the cusps should be separated along these oblique lines and any attempt to punch a hole or cut into the periphery of the stenosis was misguided and was bound to fail. I was moreover impressed with Evarts Graham's approach via the left atrial appendage and this I used. Access to the valve was easy and the cusps could be separated along the two lines of fusion by simple finger pressure. In certain cases, one had to use some form of instrument and many were designed. I used a simple knife with complete success dozens of times.

It is rarely that one achieves total understanding and success and it remained to Zimmerman to teach us more about the mitral valve. A conception of a simple oblique disposition (Fig. 5) was inadequate and could have resulted in cutting across one or both cusps. The fusion of the cusps was in a horseshoe-shaped manner and the line of separation had to follow this (Fig. 6). Simple finger separation often achieved this, but any deliberate division, especially at an open operation, had to follow this disposition.

Quite early in the operation came the Tubbs dilator. It was introduced via a small opening in the apex of the left ventricle and proved a boon to surgeons and patients alike.

Many thousands of closed mitral valvotomies were done, but a generation

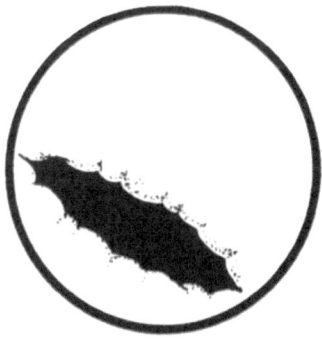

Fig. 5. Early conception of disposition of fused valves in mitral stenosis.

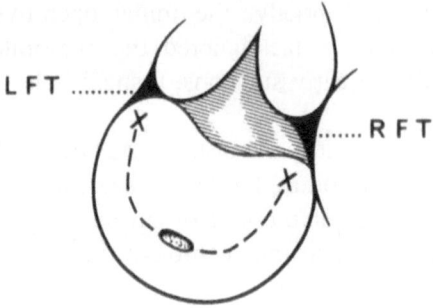

Fig. 6. Zimmermann's description of disposition of fused cusps in mitral stenosis.

is growing up that knows it not. I do not wish to discuss the merits of open versus closed mitral valvotomy, but will merely say that I and many others have had excellent results from the closed operation. I have conferred a complete cure on many patients who are fit and well with no evidence of recurrence after 25–30 years.

172

CLARENCE CRAFOORD

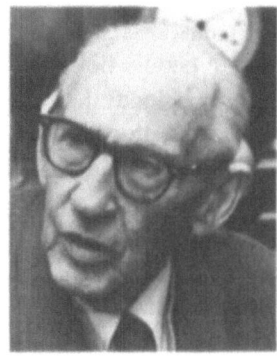

Clarence Crafoord, born in Sweden in 1899, was thoracic surgeon at Stockholm's Karolinska Hospital and chairman of the Department of Thoracic Surgery from 1957 till 1966. In 1945, he successfully pioneered the surgical treatment of coarctation of the aorta, paving the road for cardiac surgery in Europe.

Personal memories of cardiac surgery and the heart-lung machine

I intend to go back more than 50 years in time, when as a young surgeon I came in close contact with postoperative thromboembolic problems and started research concerning the various causes of these complications. At that time, I already had knowledge of Howell's and McLean's work concerning heparin, which later tremendously influenced the development within the cardiological and vascular area.

In 1927, my interest in this respect increased very much because that year I performed embolectomy in a few life-threatening cases of massive lung embolism. Two of the patients survived. Working together with Professor Jorpes, we started to assess the nature of Howell's heparin and its chemical structure in order to produce it for clinical use. Thanks to Professor Jorpes and the pharmaceutical firm Vitrum, this work had in the first part of the 1930s already progressed so far that we had available a heparin compound that we could use in repeated doses intravenously six times in 24 hours. We gave the first dose a few hours postoperatively and continued for a few days. The dosage was chosen in such a way that the coagulation time was increased to about the same extent during the whole treatment. This treatment enormously decreased the risk of thromboembolic complications in threatened cases.

We thought that oxygenation of the blood outside the body would be possible with the aid of heparin. Development of an apparatus was started in order to produce a sufficient amount of oxygenated blood in experimental animals to avoid brain damage during the time an intracardiac operation would take.

In the early part of this period, we did not consider it a realistic possibility that sufficient blood could ever be oxygenated in a machine outside a body to maintain the whole body with oxygenated blood. However, no blood should be permitted to circulate the heart and lungs during open cardiac procedures. We tried therefore to construct a machine in which so much blood could be artificially oxygenated that it would be sufficient for a prolonged survival of the brain, the organ that in all mammals least tolerates a lack of oxygen. In this way the total flow of blood to the heart and lungs and from these organs could be blocked. A part of it could be oxygenated and distributed to the brain and, in the meantime, the heart could perhaps be opened and the operation performed inside this organ.

Eventually the oxygenator was sufficiently improved to permit survival of dogs from which all venous blood was taken out before it entered the heart and was directed back to the arterial side, with the exception of the amount directed to the oxygenating machine and from there to the brain of the dog. The heart was opened and manipulated for up to 20–30 minutes with survival of the dog, as described by my co-worker Viking Olov Björk in his thesis of 1949.

During the experimental work in the end of the thirties and in the first part of the fourties, I had many times to cross-clamp the aorta above the ductus ligament. When I tried to change the original operation technique of Gross in his first ductus cases, with ligation of the ductus, to division of that vessel and, if necessary, suturing the openings in the aorta and the pulmonary artery, it was sometimes necessary to clamp the aorta just peripheral to the left subclavian artery. This made one think of the possibility to correct another congenital malformation, that is, coarctation of the aorta. I discussed the possibilities, both the diagnostic and therapeutic, with my medical and my radiological colleagues. So it happened that two cases of coarctation of the aorta were referred to us in 1944 and they were both operated upon with successful outcome, the first on 19 October and the second on 31 October 1944. In both cases the aorta was resected together with the coarctation and sutured end to end. These two cases happened to be the first two operated upon in this manner in the world.

The blood-oxygenating machine described in Björk's thesis was very much improved upon in the very end of 1949 and the beginning of 1950 by the hard work of the experimental engineers at the big AGA factory in Stockholm, Emil Anderson and after his death P. A. Åstradsson, and my assistant Åke Senning, now Professor of Surgery in Zürich. Both in size and in principle, this machine was continuously improved upon.

'What has all this to do with an Einthoven meeting on cardiology?' you may ask. In my opinion, the development within the surgical treatment of the circulatory system has been of vast importance for the evolution, not only of clinical cardiology, but also of invasive and the later-developed noninvasive diagnostic means in conjunction with refined X-ray methods. It has gradually widened the scope of cardiological diagnostic possibilities and surgical intra-cardiac treatment.

This research was much stimulated by the close and frequent exchange of experience between my friend John Gibbon, Jr., in Philadelphia, and myself. With his heart–lung machine, he performed the first reported and successful intracardiac operation. The work of the heart and the lungs in the patient was replaced for half an hour in a case of big atrial septal defect that was repaired in the summer of 1953. As Gibbon had neither the means nor possibilities of perfecting his heart–lung machine in the way he wished, he gave it to John Kirklin in the Mayo Clinics to be perfected by the experimental engineering department there.

During the same period, together with my co-workers on both the surgical and the experimental engineering sides, I advanced so far that we tried surgical repair in a few human cases of more complicated congenital intracardiac malformations, but without success, due to pulmonary hypertension. It was not until 1954 that we had our first success, the second case in the world literature. It was a case of myxoma in the left auricle, which was diagnosed preoperatively and operated upon with survival. The heart–lung machine took over the work of the patient's heart and lungs for 27 minutes, the time necessary for the intracardiac operation which was performed under induced ventricular fibrillation. This patient is still in good health.

Another development of extreme importance for progress of intrathoracic surgery, as well as cardiology, was the introduction and perfection of machinery for artificial breathing of the same effectiveness as normal respiratory function. I do not believe that it is possible to come any further still in this field than we are at the present.

However, in relation to artificial oxygenation outside the body with the help of heparin, which has also been of decisive importance for the development of cardiology, I think we have a lot to gain. In many respects this is already shown by my former assistant Per Olsson and his co-workers, working with heparinized surfaces of various plastic and other materials. The machinery for dialysis has been markedly improved and it is to be hoped that it will be possible to eliminate entirely the untoward effect on the blood that passes through a 'heart–lung machine.'

If such an improvement could be made, the time limit that we now have for the use of a heart–lung machine could practically be discarded. In acute failure, the function of a heart could be taken over for many days in succession, while during this period, the heart recovers with normal oxygenation of the blood. This would open up the road toward a completely new area of development with far-reaching consequences for cardiology as well as cardiac surgery.

PART FOUR

Einthoven Lecture

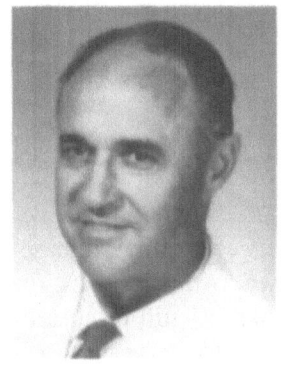

ARTHUR C. GUYTON

Arthur C. Guyton, who delivered the Einthoven Lecture, trained for surgery at Massachusetts General Hospital, where he contracted paralytic poliomyelitis. He invented several aids for the handicapped and was one of the founders of the University of Mississippi Medical Center, to which he has been attached as professor of physiology and biophysics. He is known for his classical textbook, his work as a teacher, and particularly for his vast and fundamental research on the control mechanisms of the circulation, both in health and disease.

Historical and modern development of cardiovascular control concepts

Though the basic landmarks in the history of cardiovascular discovery are well known by everyone in medicine – the elegant description of the large vascular system by Galen, the discovery of the circulation of blood by Harvey, and the first measurement of arterial pressure by Hales – on the other hand, the history of cardiovascular control concepts is fragmentary. But there is a reason for this. Most cardiovascular investigators have been interested in only one part of the circulation at a time – the heart, the arteries, the capillaries, the nervous reflexes, or the veins – so that only a few attempts have been made to put all parts of the system into perspective and to make the system work as a functioning unit.

It will be my purpose to review very briefly that portion of cardiovascular research history that does pertain specifically to cardiovascular control and then to survey recent research attempts, including our own, to solve some of the dilemmas inherited from our historical perspective. However, because of the brevity of this lecture, I would like to commend to those of you who are interested in more historical detail the excellent treatise on this subject entitled *Circulation of the Blood, Men and Ideas,* edited by Fishman and Richards, and containing articles especially pertinent to my topic by André Cournand, William Hamilton, Dickinson Richards, Eugene Landis, Corneille Heymans, Bjorn Folkow, George Pickering, and Homer Smith.

THE HISTORICAL PERSPECTIVE

Cardiovascular control can be divided into four major subdivisions, the control of (a) arterial pressure, (b) blood volume, (c) cardiac output, and (d) blood

H.A. Snellen, A.J. Dunning, A.C. Arntzenius (eds.) History and Perspectives of Cardiology, 179–201.

flow in the local tissue areas. Let us discuss each of these and also see how they fit together.

History of arterial pressure control

The first major advance in our understanding of arterial pressure control came with the studies of Bright in 1836 on the relationship between kidney disease and hypertension. From the very outset, Bright outlined two of the major concepts of arterial pressure control and hypertension that are still discussed today when he wrote '... the two most ready solutions [for hypertension] appear to be, either that the altered quality of the blood afford irregular and unwonted stimulus to the organ [heart] immediately; or that it so affects the minute and capillary circulation, as to render greater action necessary to force the blood through the distant sub-divisions of the vascular system.' Thus, Bright suggested that hypertension perhaps results from either increased activity of the heart or increased total peripheral resistance and that some abnormality of kidney function leads to one or both of these. The experimental demonstration by Goldblatt in 1934, followed by the characterization of the renin–angiotensin system by Page and his colleagues and Braun-Menéndez and his colleagues in 1939, provided especially strong support for the idea that arterial pressure is controlled by changes in total peripheral resistance.

But also on the horizon was the spector of nervous control of arterial pressure, accelerated especially by the claims of Koch and Meis in 1929, and of Heymans and Bouchaert in 1934, that denervation of the peripheral baroreceptors will cause chronic hypertension. Therefore, perhaps the basic regulator of arterial pressure was not the peripheral vascular system, not the heart, but instead the nervous system that in turn affected all of these peripheral organs; thus, another theory of arterial pressure regulation.

Also, in the background was still a fourth theory, that arterial pressure increases when the blood volume increases and decreases when volume falls. Throughout history it has never been doubted that diminished blood volume can decrease arterial pressure. Yet, Traube's suggestion in 1871 that hypertension might result from excess volume has been considered by hypertension scholars to have been a very naive concept, mainly because most hypertensive patients do not have increased blood volumes. Yet, naive or not, how was it possible to explain that many if not most patients with hypertension could be beneficially treated by volume depletion procedures – by diuretics or salt restriction? Thus, we come to the 1950s and, to some extent, even to the present time: How is arterial pressure controlled? By cardiogenic mechanisms? By changes in total peripheral resistance? By changes in nervous signals to the circulation? By changes in blood volume?

180

History of blood volume control

The basic problem in blood volume control has always been to understand the intricate balancing act between the control of salt and water intake and of renal output. One of the most significant advances in this understanding came in 1949 when Selkurt and his co-workers quantitated the relationship between arterial pressure and renal excretion of salt and water. They found, and this was corrborated almost immediately by many others, that an increase in arterial pressure has a drastic effect to increase the output of both salt and water, which is known as *pressure natriuresis* and *pressure diuresis*. Therefore, all other factors being equal, an increase in arterial pressure will cause excessive loss of fluid through the kidneys and consequent decrease in the body fluid volume.

Also, especially important in the history of blood volume control was the demonstration by Gauer and his colleagues in 1951 that an increase in central venous pressure elicits a nervous reflex that increases the urinary output; likewise, a decrease in central venous pressure causes volume retention by the kidneys. This study, and many subsequent studies on the same phenomenon, formed the basis for a widely accepted theory of blood volume control, namely, that the blood volume is regulated by nervous reflexes from the atria. However, two problems with this theory soon surfaced: first, the blood volume is regulated quite adequately even when the nerves to the heart are sectioned, such as following heart transplant operations; and, second, if the stretch receptors of the atria are like other stretch receptors of the vascular walls (the baroreceptors for instance), they adapt in one to three days and therefore cannot be used for long-term regulation of volume.

Thus, in the 1950s and at the beginning of the 1960s, our understanding of blood volume regulation was still only fragmentary. Most importantly, the overall control of fluid volume by the kidneys was believed to be based mainly on a reflex mechanism, even though elimination of this reflex caused very little change in volume regulation.

History of cardiac output regulation

Because it is the heart that pumps the blood, most of the history of cardiac output control has centered around the heart and heart mechanisms. Fick, in 1867, laid the groundwork for understanding the pumping action of the heart when he described the relationship between muscle length and force of muscle contraction – that, within physiological limits, an increase in the initial length of muscle causes a corresponding increase in strength of contraction. But it remained for Frank (1895) to apply this principle to the heart when he pointed out that the greater the degree of filling of a heart, the greater also is the pressure attained during systolic contraction. Soon thereafter, Starling (1918) formulated his 'Law of the Heart' which, simply stated, is the following: Within physiological limits, the heart pumps whatever amount of blood flows into the right atrium and does so without a significant rise in right atrial pressure. For about 40 years thereafter, it was assumed that the cardiac output is controlled mainly by 'venous return' – that is, that mechanisms in the peripheral circulation determine the rate of blood flow into the heart and that this in turn determines the cardiac output.

But in the 1950s, new studies were forthcoming on nervous control of the heart, especially by Rushmer and his colleagues (1959), and these were impressive enough that it soon became widely held that the venous return concept of control was mainly dead and that the nervous system, in all its wisdom, was the real controller of cardiac output. This view was held even in the 1960s, when Hamilton and Richards wrote in 1964: 'It is now held that in the normal animal, as distinguished from the usual physiologist's preparation, the venous return is always ample to fill the heart and is hence not a key to the regulation of cardiac output. On the other hand, the pumping action of the heart is regulated reflexly to maintain the arterial pressure within physiological limits despite the changes in flow.' But this statement did not reckon with the coming of the heart transplant, for when hearts began to be transplanted and they had no nervous control, nevertheless, this procedure had no perceptible effect on the normal control of either cardiac output or arterial pressure. So, was the venous return theory of cardiac output regulation dead after all?

History of local tissue control of blood flow

Cardiac output control is always indelibly linked to blood flow control in the local tissues because the sum of all tissue flow must equal the cardiac output. It has long been known that increased activity in tissues increases the local blood flow, this is especially so in muscles where the activity can increase for a few seconds at a time as much as 100-fold and the local blood flow as much as 20-fold. But what is it that causes the increased flow?

As early as 1879, Roy and Brown suggested that the local concentration of oxygen in the tissues might be one of the factors that controls the flow. This same concept was developed further by Krogh (1919), who observed that many dormant blood vessels open up during muscle activity, which led him to assume, mainly theoretically, that this resulted in part from decreased tissue oxygen.

Through the years it has also been suggested that other factors instead of,

182

or in addition to, oxygen might be principal controllers of local blood flow during increased tissue activity – such factors as carbon dioxide, hydrogen ions, histamine, potassium ions, bradykinin, serotonin, and, more recently, adenosine and ATP. Especially strong support has been advanced in the past few years for a mechanism that goes like this (Berne 1974): Increased tissue activity decreases the tissue oxygen supply and this in turn causes adenosine to be released from the hypoxic tissue cells. The adenosine in turn dilates the local blood vessels so that the tissue oxygen level now returns to a normal level. But there are problems with this mechanism: mainly a difficulty to prove that enough adenosine can be released from the tissues to cause long-term vasodilatation in such conditions as circulatory shock or femoral artery occlusion, both of which cause intense local vasodilatation.

But, whatever the mechanism, it is clear that either an increase in tissue activity or a decrease in delivery of oxygen to the tissues will lead to marked increase in local tissue blood flow. In this way, an increase in tissue metabolism in widespread areas of the body can easily lead to increased blood flow through the systemic circulation and thence back to the heart, thus also leading to increased cardiac output.

A special feature of essentially all mechanisms of local tissue blood flow control is that they lead to the phenomenon called *autoregulation*. That is, when the arterial pressure rises and the tissue blood flow increases as a result, this automatically causes peripheral arteriolar constriction that decreases the flow back toward normal. Therefore, an increase in arterial pressure does not necessarily increase the tissue blood flow very much. Later in this paper we shall see that one of the important theories of hypertension proposes that the increase in total peripheral resistance seen in much hypertension results from this autoregulation phenomenon.

SOME OF THE DILEMMAS OF CARDIOVASCULAR CONTROL AT THE BEGINNING OF THE MODERN ERA

By 1950, and even more so by 1960, the function of most individual parts of the circulation had been studied in depth, but the way in which all these parts function together to provide a controlled circulation was still elusive. Some of the major dilemmas were the following:

1) Even into the 1960s, it was believed by most physiologists that cardiac output is controlled mainly by nervous signals to the heart. But, as pointed out earlier, with the coming of the heart transplant era, as well as in consequence of many other studies, it was soon clear that cardiac output is controlled almost equally as well in the absence of nervous signals to the heart as when they are present – except at the extremes of cardiac output requirement.

2) The heart transplant experience also disproved the idea that reflexes are of major importance for the long-term control of blood volume, because either transplantation of the heart or denervation of the cardiac receptors in other ways did not materially change the blood volume.

3) The most widely held theory of arterial pressure control was that pressure is controlled almost entirely by changes in total peripheral resistance. But measurements in patients with decreases in total peripheral resistance to as little as one-half normal – such as in patients with chronic arteriovenous shunts, in beriberi, thyrotoxicosis, and anemia – all showed no correlation between the abnormal total peripheral resistance and the arterial pressure level. How could these observations be true if total peripheral resistance were the major factor controlling the long-term level of arterial pressure? But, on the other hand, if changes in total peripheral resistance are not the long-term controller of arterial pressure, why is it that one almost always finds very high total peripheral resistance in patients with essential hypertension? Thus, probably the greatest dilemma of all was the conflict between (a) the supposition by most pressure control enthusiasts that arterial pressure is controlled almost entirely by total peripheral resistance, and (b) the opposing proposition put forth by those interested in cardiac output control that the long-term level of cardiac output is mainly controlled by changes in total peripheral resistance. Unfortunately, a decrease in total peripheral resistance increases the cardiac output but decreases the arterial pressure, a dichotomy that is not found to occur in most functional states of the circulation.

Therefore, there remained many missing links.

ATTEMPTS TO RESOLVE THE DILEMMAS

Over the past 25 years, the major goal of our laboratory has been to develop an overall analysis of cardiovascular regulation. Therefore, in the following sections, I will refer to our own efforts to solve some of these dilemmas, though of course many others have played equally as important roles.

Is cardiac output controlled by heart activity or by peripheral circulatory factors?

In the early 1950s, Sarnoff and his colleagues (1955) restudied the Frank–Starling 'Law of the Heart,' especially adding quantitative data that was necessary to understand its importance as a circulatory control mechanism. In essence, they demonstrated that very slight increases in the right atrial input pressure to the heart can even normally increase the cardiac output severalfold. We in our laboratory corroborated Sarnoff's results and also added two other bits of data that were necessary to understand the overall importance of this law of the heart:

First, even under normal resting conditions, the heart is capable of pumping two to three times as much blood as it normally pumps without being stimulated by the nerves or any other extracardiac factor; all that is required is an increase in the flow of blood into the right atrium (Guyton 1963; Bishop 1964). Thus, the heart has 100% – 200% *cardiac output reserve* even under normal resting pumping conditions.

Second, when the heart rate is increased to approximately two times normal by electrical pacing signals applied to the internal wall of the right atrium, the pumping capacity of the heart increases about 50% if the right atrial pressure is experimentally maintained at a constant pressure level. Yet, when the same experiment is performed under normal physiological conditions, without resorting to special procedures to maintain a constant right atrial pressure, instead of the cardiac output increasing 50%, it does not increase at all. Instead, the right atrial pressure decreases and the veins entering the thoracic cavity collapse even more than normally, thus causing a blood-flow waterfall into the heart (Sugimoto 1966; Cowley 1971). Thus it was immediately clear that increasing the pumping capacity of the heart is not a sufficient cause by itself to increase the cardiac output.

Quantification of the roles of the heart and of the peripheral circulation for the control of cardiac output. In still other experiments, we studied separately and quantitatively (a) the capability of the heart to pump blood, and (b) the

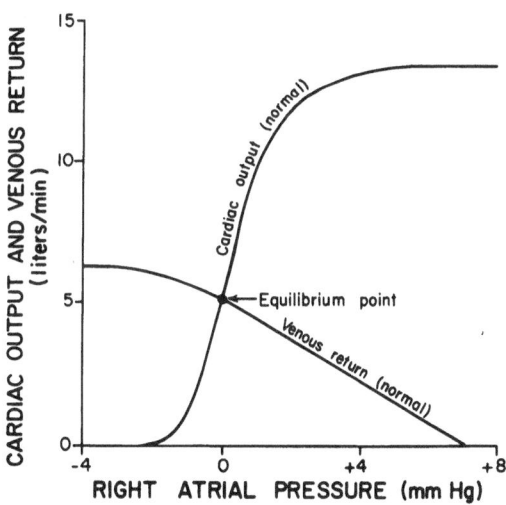

Fig. 1. Equating the normal cardiac output curve with the normal venous return curve. The 'equilibrium point' defines the normal operating level of cardiac output. (Reprinted from Guyton et al., *Cardiac output and its control.* Philadelphia: WB Saunders, 1973.)

185

capability of the blood to flow from the peripheral circulation into the heart (Guyton 1955, 1963). These two separate effects were displayed in the form of (a) cardiac output curves depicting the ability of the heart to pump, and (b) venous return curves depicting the ability of blood to flow from the systemic circulation back to the heart. The 'resting' cardiac output curve and the 'resting' venous return curve for the normal human being, as extrapolated from data obtained in dogs, are illustrated in Figure 1. Since venous return, except for a few beats of the heart at a time, must equal the cardiac output, the actual operating cardiac output level is depicted by the point at which the venous return and cardiac output curves cross, labeled in the figure 'equilibrium point.' Note especially that the cardiac output curve has a plateau at *high atrial pressures* because the heart reaches its physiological pumping limit. On the other hand, the venous return curve reaches a plateau at very low atrial pressures, when the pressure falls below atmospheric pressure (below zero), because atmospheric pressure pressing on the extrathoracic veins then causes them to collapse and to impede venous flow. But note also that the level of the cardiac output plateau is much higher than the actual cardiac output (where the two curves cross), while the plateau of the venous return curve is only slightly higher. Furthermore, one can easily see that increasing the entire level of the cardiac output curve could have almost no effect on the point at which this curve crosses the venous return curve and therefore could have almost no effect on cardiac output. For this reason, increasing the level of heart-pumping activity is not a significant mechanism for increasing the cardiac output under otherwise normal resting conditions. On the other hand, it is equally clear that increasing the overall level of the venous return curve would be highly beneficial in increasing the cardiac output. Therefore, we can quickly come to the conclusion that it is mainly peripheral vascular factors that control the normal variations in cardiac output and that the heart merely acts as an automatic relay pumping station, subserving the needs of the peripheral circulation but not dictating these needs.

The mechanism for increasing cardiac output during circulatory stress, such as during muscle activity. During circulatory stress, several circulatory factors affect both the venous return curve and the cardiac output curve. For instance, Figure 2 illustrates four different stages during the onset of moderate exercise. The cardiac output increases progressively from point A to point B, then to point C, and finally to point D. The increase to point B results from compression of the veins by the contracting muscles. This shifts the venous return curve to the long-dashed curve and thereby translocates blood toward the heart; the new curve equates with the cardiac output curve at point B, thus instantaneously increasing the cardiac output a slight amount at the very onset of exercise. Next, the circulation begins to be stimulated by the

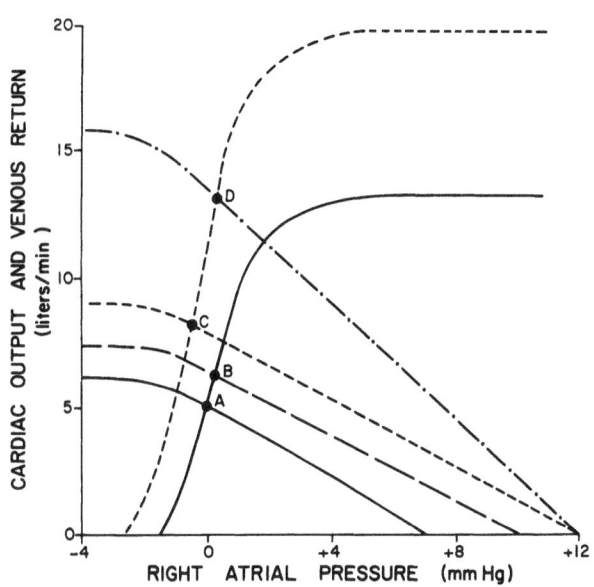

Fig. 2. Graphical analysis of the changes in cardiac output at various time intervals following the onset of moderate exercise. (Reprinted from Guyton et al., *Cardiac output and its regulation.* Philadelphia: WB Saunders, 1973)

sympathetic nervous system; this contracts the capacitance vessels throughout the circulation and also stimulates the heart, thereby increasing the venous return curve still further to the short-dashed curve and also increasing the output curve to the corresponding short-dashed curve. These two curves now equate with each other at point C, and the cardiac output rises still more. But the major effect to increase the cardiac output results from vasodilatation in the active muscles. This rotates the venous return curve up to the dot-dashed curve, which in turn equates with the cardiac output curve of the sympathetically stimulated heart at point D.

Thus, the analysis of Figure 2 illustrates that essentially all of the increase in cardiac output in this instance resulted from changes in the venous return curve – changes caused by altered parameters of blood flow through the peripheral circulation – and not from the changes in pumping activity by the heart. However, it is equally clear that, if still more increase in cardiac output had been required, then the sympathetic stimulation of cardiac pumping would have been required to prevent heart failure. Thus, nervous stimulation of the heart mainly provides an overload-pumping capacity for the heart, but it does not play a significant role in control of cardiac output at the usual levels of daily life.

Effect of total peripheral resistance on the long-term control of cardiac output.
From the literature, I have collected data relating total peripheral resistance to

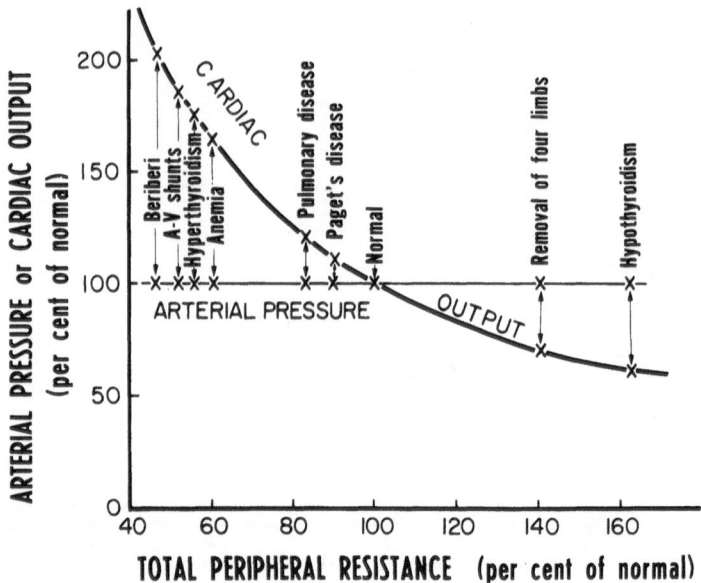

Fig. 3. Relationship between (a) total peripheral resistance and the long-term level of cardiac output, and (b) total peripheral resistance and the long-term level of arterial pressure, illustrating an inverse effect of total peripheral resistance on cardiac output but no effect on the arterial pressure. (Reprinted from Guyton, *Arterial pressure and hypertension.* Philadelphia: WB Saunders, in press 1980.)

both the long-term level of cardiac output and the long-term level of arterial pressure. These relationships are illustrated in Figure 3 (Guyton 1980). Among the conditions that decrease the total peripheral resistance are arteriovenous shunt, beriberi, anemia, Paget's disease, and hyperthyroidism. And two conditions that increase the total peripheral resistance are hypothyroidism and removal of the four limbs. In none of these instances is the arterial pressure known to change from the normal, but, in all, the long-term cardiac output level is inversely proportional to the change in total peripheral resistance in accord with the following equation:

$$\text{cardiac output} = \frac{\text{arterial pressure}}{\text{total peripheral resistance}}$$

The reason for this inverse relationship is simply that, if the arterial pressure does not change from normal, then any factor that causes a long-term decrease in the total peripheral resistance will automatically increase the flow of blood from the arteries into the right atrium and therefore a corresponding increase in cardiac output as well.

Thus, it is the cardiac output that is controlled by long-term changes in total peripheral resistance, not the arterial pressure.

188

Control of local blood flow

In the above discussion, it was pointed out that the major cause of the increased cardiac output during exercise is the great decrease in resistance to blood flow through the muscle. And this results from increased activity in the muscles, an effect that also occurs in almost any tissue of the body when its activity increases.

However, our knowledge of local blood flow control during increased activity has advanced hardly at all in the last 15 years. The vast majority of physiologists still believe that vasodilator substances released by active tissues cause local vasodilatation and increased flow. Also, a large amount of qualitative evidence favors such a mechanism. The vasodilator agent most often implicated is adenosine, especially in the coronary circulation where this has been studied most extensively (Berne 1974). Yet, full quantitative proof of this is still elusive.

Thus, the search for the different vasodilator factors that control local blood flow has now been going on for more than 50 years, and still the final answer is not clear. Therefore, still another possibility for the increased blood flow during activity should also be considered: that tissue activity diminishes one or more vasoconstrictor substances and in this way allows passive vasodilatation. One such vasoconstrictor is oxygen. Figure 4 illustrates the effect on blood flow in the hindlimb of the dog caused by progressive decrease in

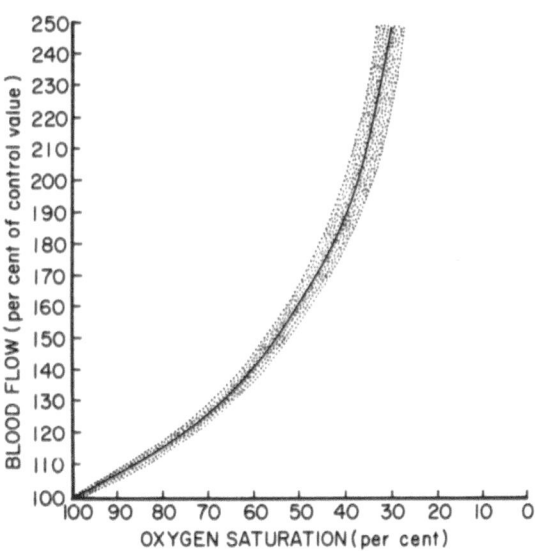

Fig. 4. Effect on blood flow in the hindlimb of the dog, caused by progressive decrease in arterial oxygen saturation. Average results from ten dogs; the shaded area represents probable errors of the means. (Drawn from data in Crawford et al. 1959.)

arterial oxygen saturation (Crawford 1959). And still other studies have shown that decreased oxygen also increases blood flow through small arteries isolated from their surrounding tissues, illustrating that even the arterial wall itself, even in the absence of surrounding tissues, relaxes when the oxygen concentration falls (Carrier 1964). Therefore, it is still possible that the principal cause of local vasodilatation during tissue activity is the increased consumption of oxygen and of other metabolic substrates by the tissues, thus reducing the availability of these to the vascular walls and thereby allowing them to dilate.

Control of arterial pressure

Is arterial pressure controlled by changing the total peripheral resistance? Let us return briefly to Figure 3, which showed the relationship between total peripheral resistance and both cardiac output and arterial pressure in a series of different clinical conditions. Note in this figure that the arterial pressure was normal in each instance despite the very abnormal total peripheral resistances. Instead, it was the cardiac output that changed, not the arterial pressure. Therefore, the data itself shows that it is untenable to suggest that changes in total peripheral resistance necessarily alter the long-term level of arterial pressure.

Yet, we also know that in almost all instances of chronic hypertension the total peripheral resistance is greatly increased, and the cardiac output only rarely increased. How can we reconcile this with the data in Figure 3? This, we will attempt to answer in the following discussions.

Experimental volume-loading hypertension. Let us first recall that Traube as long ago as 1871 suggested that renal hypertension results from retention of fluid in the body. But let us also recall that most authorities in hypertension research have considered this to be a very naive thought. Was it so naive after all?

Because many phenomena of both experimental and clinical hypertension could not be explained on the basis of primary increases in total peripheral resistance, and because there was no ready explanation for the inability of primary increases in total peripheral resistance to cause hypertension in many clinical conditions, as illustrated in Figure 3, several different research workers in the early 1960s came to an almost simultaneous conclusion that volume does indeed play an almost indispensible role in the long-term control of arterial pressure – Borst (1963) in Holland, Ledingham (1963, 1964) in England, and Conway (1966) and ourselves (Guyton 1961; Langston 1963) in the United States. The concept of all of these investigators was that an increase in volume will eventually increase the arterial pressure, that this will then increase the blood flow through the tissues, and the blood flow through the tissues will cause a secondary increase in total peripheral resistance to return the total tissue blood flow and cardiac output nearly back to normal. In other words, this theory suggests that the increase in total peripheral resistance in hypertension is secondary, caused by the blood flow autoregulation phenomenon and that it is not a primary factor in the initial development of at least some types of hypertension.

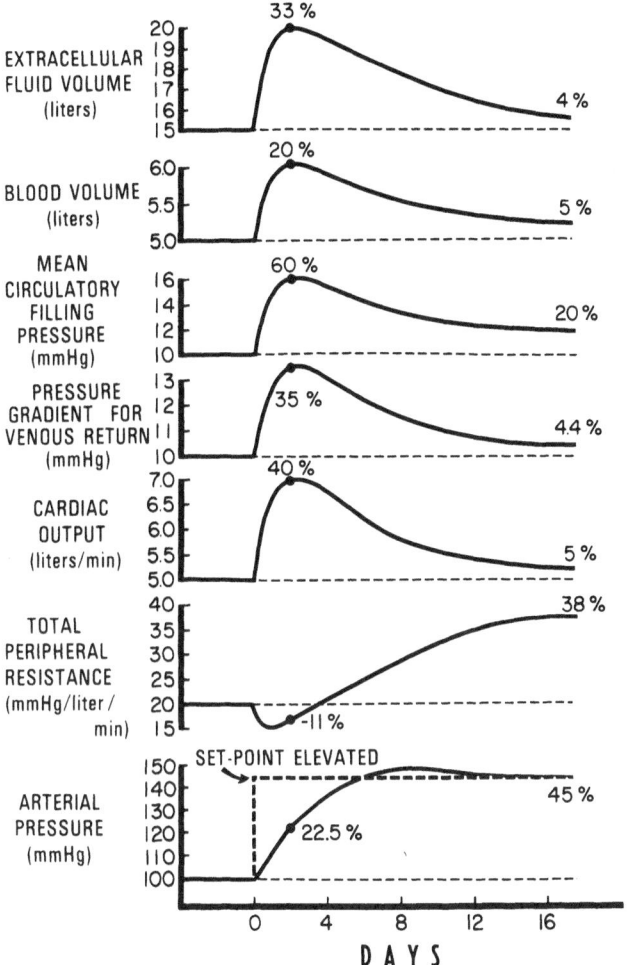

Fig. 5. Average composite changes in important circulatory variables during the onset of chronic volume-loading hypertension, caused by reducing the kidney mass to approximately 30% of normal and then infusing isotonic saline continuously for several weeks at a sodium intake level approximately five times normal. (Reprinted from Guyton, *Arterial pressure and hypertension.* Philadelphia: WB Saunders, in press 1980.)

191

Yet, experimental proof for this was very difficult to find because even a slight rise in volume and arterial pressure causes rapid pressure diuresis and natriuresis, so that both the excess volume and the increased pressure are automatically corrected as rapidly as one attempts to increase the volume. To obviate this difficulty, we began a series of experiments in the early 1960s in which most of the kidney mass of dogs was first removed so that the kidneys could not excrete water and salt very rapidly. Then it became possible to cause increases in blood volume and in arterial pressure lasting for days or weeks. The results of these experiments are summarized in Figure 5, which gives a composite of many of our results over the past 18 years (Langston 1963; Douglas 1964; Coleman 1969; Granger 1969; Guyton 1967, 1969, 1972, 1974; Cowley 1975; DeClue 1978; Manning 1979).

In the composite experiment illustrated in Figure 5, one kidney and the two poles of the opposite kidney of a dog had already been removed, leaving only the central portion of one kidney. Then, at zero days, the intake of salt and water was increased to approximately five times normal and maintained at this level for the remainder of the experiment. All of the variables that were directly related to the volume load increased rapidly on the very first day and reached a peak in two to three days; these included blood volume, extracellular fluid volume, cardiac output, mean circulatory filling pressure, and pressure gradient for venous return. However, by the end of two to three weeks, all of these had returned almost to normal – but not quite so.

On the other hand, the changes in total peripheral resistance were quite different. During the first few days this actually decreased, reaching a nadir approximately 25% *below* normal during the first day. But then the total peripheral resistance began to rise, and by the end of two to three weeks it was elevated to an average of about 38% *above* normal when all the other variables related directly to volume had already returned almost to normal.

But, when did the arterial pressure rise? The answer is: from the very beginning of the experiment, paralleling the early rise in the volume and cardiac output. Furthermore, most of the increase in arterial pressure occurred before the total peripheral resistance rose even above the original control level. And it was only during the latter days of the experiment that the volume factors and cardiac output returned almost to normal while the total peripheral resistance increased – all of this with the arterial pressure still remaining elevated.

Thus, in these experiments the increase in total peripheral resistance lagged behind the increase in arterial pressure. It did not precede nor even parallel it. This is exactly what one would expect if the increase in total peripheral resistance were a secondary effect caused by autoregulation, and it is not at all the effect that would have occurred if the increase in total peripheral resistance had been primary and the rise in arterial pressure secondary.

Thus, these experiments, as well as experiments from Ledingham's laboratory (1963, 1964) and clinical experiences reported especially by Birkenhager and Schalekämp (1976) and their colleagues, have all suggested that there is in reality such a thing as volume-loading hypertension and that in this type of hypertension the increase in total peripheral resistance is a secondary phenomenon, almost certainly resulting from the autoregulation mechanism.

How much volume increase is required to cause hypertension? Please note very carefully the extracellular fluid volume, blood volume, and cardiac output toward the end of the experiment in Figure 5. None of these at that time were still elevated above the control level more than a few percent. Yet, there is all the reason in the world to believe that these slight increases in volume and cardiac output were necessary to sustain the elevated pressure. The reason for believing this was very simple: within 24–72 h after the excess salt and water intake was canceled, the arterial pressure returned to normal.

Role of the kidney in hypertension – the renal function curve and the principle of infinite gain. One of the keys to the success of the volume-loading hypertension experiment was the initial reduction of the kidney mass. Because of this, the kidney would not excrete the increased salt and water load as rapidly as it was given to the animal, and true volume overloads could then be maintained for long periods. On the other hand, when the kidneys were normal, volume overloads could not be maintained, and the maximum that we could increase the arterial pressure with salt and water loading was 4–8 mmHg. Therefore, it immediately became clear to us that the normal kidneys have a tremendous capacity for excreting volume overloads and for doing so within a few minutes to a few hours, thereby almost never allowing the arterial pressure to rise significantly as a result of volume overload.

To study the phenomenon of volume-loading hypertension quantitatively we measured what we have called the 'chronic volume-loading renal function curve.' Several different ones of these curves are illustrated in Figure 6, both for the normal kidneys and for different abnormal states of kidney function. Such curves are measured by infusing saline into the animal continuously but at progressively greater levels every two days. Within approximately 24 h after each infusion rate increase, the animal's urinary output rises to equal the intake. Therefore, we can determine the steady-state relationship between arterial pressure and urinary output at the end of each two-day period of infusion. The curve for the normal animal (labeled 'normal') illustrates that the urinary output of sodium (and of water as well) can increase tremendously with almost no increase in pressure.

But now note the abnormal renal function curves. Such abnormalities can result from pathology of the kidneys or from abnormal stimulation of the kidneys by such factors as angiotensin, aldosterone, or nervous stimulation. In general, all of these factors tend to shift the renal function curve toward a higher pressure level, but they also often change the characteristics of the renal function curve as well.

Now, note the horizontal line through the curves in Figure 6 labeled 'normal intake.' This crosses the normal renal function curve at point A. One can readily see that if the pressure rises higher than the pressure level of point A, the output of salt will become far greater than the intake because of the pressure natriuresis mechanism, and the output of water will also increase simultaneously because of the pressure diuresis phenomenon. Consequently, over a period of hours or days, loss of salt and water will cause the arterial pressure to fall exactly back to point A, where the renal function curve and the intake line cross each other. Since this mechanism represents a negative feedback control system and since the pressure always returns exactly to the point of crossing of the two curves, this mechanism for control of arterial pressure has *infinite* feedback gain. This is an extremely important characteristic of this control system because it allows this system to dominate all the other pressure control systems (Guyton 1972, 1974).

However, note that the infinite gain principle holds only so long as neither the intake level nor the renal function curve changes. But if some factor does change either the intake level or the renal function curve, then the new crossing point of the function curve with the intake line becomes the pressure control level, and the kidney-volume-pressure feedback control system will now automatically control the arterial pressure at this new 'set-point' level.

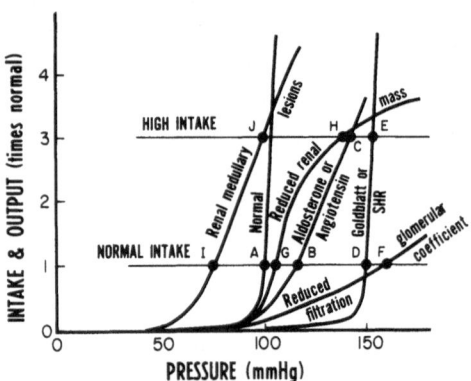

Fig. 6. The normal renal function curve and five abnormal function curves caused by (1) reduced renal mass, (2) aldosterone or angiotensin infusion, (3) Goldblatt clamps on both renal arteries or spontaneous hypertension, (4) reduced glomerular filtration coefficient, and (5) renal medullary lesions. Note also the points where the different function curves cross the two different levels of salt intake. These points of crossing represent the levels at which the arterial pressure will be regulated for each given combination. (Reprinted from Guyton, *Arterial pressure and hypertension*. Philadelphia: WB Saunders, in press 1980.)

194

The only way to change the pressure to still a new level is to change once again either the intake level or the renal function curve. Thus, in Figure 6, when aldosterone is infused into an animal the renal function curve rotates to the right, and the arterial pressure becomes controlled at point B with a new pressure level of 116 mmHg. In the animal with spontaneous hypertension and with normal intake, the pressure becomes controlled at point D with a pressure of 150 mmHg. And, when the kidney mass has been reduced to about 30% of normal and the salt intake increased to the level of the 'high intake' line in Figure 6, the arterial pressure becomes controlled at point H with a pressure of 140 mmHg.

How do vasoconstrictor factors, hormonal or nervous, increase the arterial pressure? In earlier discussions of this paper, it has already been pointed out that primary changes in total peripheral resistance resulting from arteriovenous shunts, beriberi, anemia, thyrotoxicosis, hypothyroidism, removal of all four limbs, or from many other causes do not affect the long-term level of arterial pressure. Yet, there is much valuable experience which shows that circulating vasoconstrictor agents such as catecholamines and angiotensin, and perhaps increased sympathetic activity as well, can all cause chronic elevation of the arterial pressure. Furthermore, these factors all increase the total peripheral resistance. Therefore, what is the difference between the increased total peripheral resistance resulting from the vasoconstrictor factors versus the increased total peripheral resistance that occurs in the primary abnormalities of the circulation listed above? The answer to this is that the catecholamines, angiotensin, and sympathetic stimulation not only constrict the peripheral systemic blood vessels, but they decrease renal output of sodium and water as well. Thus, they shift the renal function curve to the right on the graph shown in Figure 6, so that the arterial pressure level then becomes much higher than before. On the other hand, all the clinical conditions discussed above that cause primary changes in total peripheral resistance without causing hypertention are different because none of them change renal function. Therefore, the difference between the two is not the change in total peripheral resistance, but instead the coincident effect of the generalized vasoconstrictor factor on renal function. Thus, the way vasoconstrictor factors cause hypertension is to depress renal excretory function, not their effect on total peripheral resistance.

Effect of vasoconstrictor factors on blood volume and cardiac output in hypertension. Most vasoconstrictor hormones, as well as sympathetic stimulation, also constrict the capacitance vessels of the circulation. At first, this increases the cardiac output and elevates the arterial pressure, but the elevated pressure again causes pressure natriuresis and pressure diuresis until the blood volume falls low enough to bring the arterial pressure back to normal. This same effect can also be demonstrated by putting tight binders on the legs of patients to constrict large varicose veins. The increase in arterial pressure that occurs is only transient.

Nevertheless, it is still important to remember that vasoconstrictors do decrease the sizes of the capacitance vessels throughout the body, because this means that less blood volume is then required to maintain the arterial pressure either at the normal blood pressure level or even at hypertensive levels. Therefore, a patient who has hypertension and who simultaneously has a vasoconstrictor factor such as renin from a diseased kidney might also have less than normal blood volume. If you will think about this for a moment, you will see that this does not in any way invalidate the importance of the kidney-volume-pressure mechanism in pressure control. And it also does not invalidate the infinite gain principle. It simply means that the presence of vasoconstrictor factors that decrease vascular capacitance and increase arteriolar resistance allows the kidney-volume-pressure mechanism to adjust both the blood volume and the cardiac output to lower levels when controlling arterial pressure than are required in the absence of the vasoconstrictor factors. Please pause and think about this for a while, because many research workers in the field of hypertension have made the error of stating that decreased blood volume and decreased cardiac output in hypertension are prima facie evidence against a volume mechanism for controlling arterial pressure. This is not true.

Control of blood volume

It is already clear that blood volume control is inextricably linked to the control of arterial pressure. Very simply, when the arterial pressure increases, the kidneys vastly increase their output of both salt and water until both volume and pressure return to normal. Likewise, it is common knowledge that when the volume falls too low, so also does the pressure fall. And renal retention of fluid then eventually returns both the blood volume and the pressure back to normal.

Therefore, there seems to be no special magic in the control of blood volume. Also, there is no special reason for controlling blood volume per se. Instead, blood volume (and extracellular fluid volume too) is really the servant of pressure control because it is mainly pressure control, not volume control, that is fundamental to proper functioning of the circulatory system.

What is the quantitative relationship between blood volume and arterial pressure? If blood volume is so important to pressure control, what is the

196

quantitative relationship between blood volume and pressure? The answer to this is twofold: Under acute conditions, the blood volume has to change a large amount to change the arterial pressure even a small amount. But, under chronic conditions, very slight changes in blood volume seem to have very marked effects on the long-term arterial pressure level. Both of these effects were illustrated by the volume-loading hypertension experiment in Figure 5. During the first few days of the hypertension, the increase in the volume required to increase the pressure was very great, but by the end of two to three weeks only about one-tenth as much volume was necessary to sustain the hypertension. Most of the reasons for these differences have now been determined. First, in the acute state, the nervous reflexes attempt to keep the arterial pressure from rising, and part of the reflex effect is to dilate the capacitance vessels of the circulation. Therefore, far more increase in blood volume is required acutely to increase the arterial pressure than is required chronically, because, chronically, essentially all of the nervous reflexes adapt and fall by the wayside. Second, still another factor that contributes to the extremely small amount of excess volume required to maintain chronic hypertension is the autoregulation phenomenon. When the peripheral arterioles constrict as a result of too much blood flow through the tissues (which is the autoregulation mechanism), this constriction increases the total peripheral resistance but also decreases the venous pressure. And, since most of the blood volume is normally in the veins, once the autoregulation mechanism has developed fully, far less volume is required to maintain the hypertensive state.

From our studies on volume-loading hypertension and also from other studies in which low volume was studied in dogs with a pathological renal

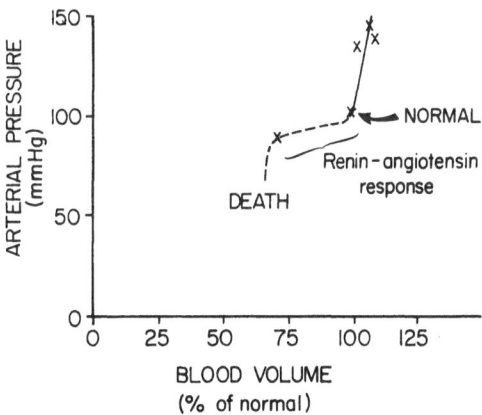

Fig. 7. A semiquantitative curve showing the relationship between blood volume and long-term arterial pressure level. (Reprinted from Guyton et al., in *Osmotic and volume regulation.* Copenhagen: Munksgaard, 1978, p 283.)

197

salt-losing syndrome, we have been able to piece together a semiquantitative curve showing the long-term relationship between blood volume and arterial pressure (Guyton 1978). This is illustrated in Figure 7. When the volume is increased to levels only slightly above normal and maintained at these levels for several weeks, the arterial pressure rises markedly. On the other hand, slight decreases in volume are not associated with marked decreases in pressure. Instead, the renin–angiotensin system becomes strongly activated, and the pressure is maintained almost at normal levels despite as much as 30% decrease in blood volume. However, we noted that the dogs whose pressures were maintained in this way by massive secretion of renin also lived precarious lives, because several of them died within minutes as a result of nothing more than fright or some other intercurrent stress to the circulation. Our initial observations, therefore, suggest that the renin–angiotensin system plays an exceedingly important role in maintaining the arterial pressure at or near normal in hypovolemic states. Were it not for this system, one would suspect that even very slight long-term hypovolemia would be associated with severe decreases in arterial pressure, which indeed does occur if a renin- or angiotensin-blocking drug is given.

In essence, therefore, all of the evidence that we can muster suggests that volume is a critical factor in arterial pressure control, especially in long-term pressure control. Also, the magnitude of the volume changes that are required to effect marked increases in arterial pressure is very slight, so slight indeed that the usual methods for measuring blood volume are only barely adequate to detect blood volumes greater than normal even in experiments of pure-volume-loading hypertension.

SUMMARY

In this paper, I have presented a very brief history of cardiovascular control concepts and especially have discussed attempts to solve some of the remaining dilemmas.

From our own studies, as well as those of others, we have been greatly impressed by the essential role that blood volume plays in long-term control of arterial pressure and also by the minuteness of the changes in volume that are required to affect drastically the long-term arterial pressure level. Furthermore, our analyses, both experimental and mathematical, have brought us to the conclusion that the kidney-volume-pressure control system is an infinite gain system that controls the arterial pressure to a very exact level so long as all of its parts function normally. Indeed, because of this infinite gain feature, only those factors that change either renal function or the intake level of salt and water can, in the long run, alter the long-term arterial pressure level.

Once the arterial pressure is controlled, then each individual tissue can control its own local blood flow by simply dilating its blood vessels in response to local needs. And many different experiments have demonstrated that increased tissue activity does invariably dilate the local vessels.

Finally, cardiac output is the sum of the flows through all the individual tissues. Therefore, the long-term level of cardiac output normally is controlled not by the heart, but by all those peripheral circulatory factors that go into controlling all the local flows.

Thus, the entire premise of circulatory control is that blood flow to the tissues is of paramount importance, and the system is so engineered to allow each tissue, in the long run, to determine its own flow. Arterial pressure control, volume control, and cardiac output control are only servants to this end.

REFERENCES

Berne RM, Rubio R (1974) Regulation of coronary blood flow. Adv Cardiol 12:303
Birkenhäger WH, Schalekamp MADH (1976) Control mechanisms in essential hypertension. Amsterdam: Elsevier
Bishop VS, Stone HL, Guyton AC (1964) Cardiac function curves in conscious dogs. Am J Physiol 206:677
Braun-Menendez E, Fasciolo JC, Leloir LF, Munoz JM (1939) La substancia hipertensora de la sangre del rinon isquemiado. Rev Soc Argent Biol 15:420
Bright R (1836) Tabular view of the morbid appearances in 100 cases connected with albuminous urine. With observations. Guy's Hosp Rep 1:380
Borst JGG, Borst-De Geus A (1963) Hypertension explained by Starling's theory of circulatory homeostasis. Lancet 1:677
Carrier O, Walker J, Guyton AC (1964) Role of oxygen in autoregulation of blood flow in isolated vessels. Am J Physiol 206:951
Coleman TG, Guyton AC (1969) Hypertension caused by salt loading in the dog. Onset transients of cardiac output and other circulatory variables. Circ Res 25:152
Conway J (1966) Hemodynamic consequences of induced changes in blood volume. Circ Res 18:190
Cowley AW Jr, Guyton AC (1971) Heart rate as a determinant of cardiac output in dogs with arteriovenous fistula. Am J Cardiol 28:321
Cowley AW Jr, Guyton AC (1975) Baroreceptor reflex effects on transient and steady-state hemodynamics of salt-loading hypertension in dogs. Circ Res 36:536
Crawford DG, Fairchild HM, Guyton AC (1959) Oxygen lack as a possible cause of reactive hyperemia. Am J Physiol 197:613
DeClue JW, Guyton AC, Cowley AW Jr, Coleman TG, Norman RA Jr, McCaa RE (1978) Subpressor angiotensin infusion, renal sodium handling, and salt-induced hypertension in the dog. Circ Res 43:503
Douglas BH, Guyton AC, Langston JB, Bishop VS (1964) Hypertension caused by salt loading. II: Fluid volume and tissue pressure changes. Am J Physiol 207:669
Fick A (1964) Untersuchungen über Muskel-Arbeit. Basel: Georg
Fishman AP, Richards DW (eds) (1964) Circulation of the blood – men and ideas. New York: Oxford University Press

Frank O (1895) Zur Dynamik des Herzmuskels. Z Biol 32:370

Gauer OH, Henry JP, Sicker HO, Wendt WE (1951) Heart and lungs as a receptor region controlling blood volume. Am J Physiol 167:786

Goldblatt H, Lynch J, Hanzai RE, Summerville WW (1934) Studies on experimental hypertension. I. The production of persistent elevation of systolic blood pressure by means of renal ischemia. J Exp Med 59:347

Granger HJ, Guyton AC (1969) Autoregulation of the total systemic circulation following destruction of the central nervous system in the dog. Circ Res 25:379.

Guyton AC (1955) Determination of cardiac output by equating venous return curves with cardiac response curves. Physiol Rev 35:123

Guyton AC (1961) Textbook of medical physiology. Philadelphia: WB Saunders, p 437

Guyton AC (1963) Circulatory physiology: cardiac output and its regulation. Philadelphia: WB Saunders

Guyton AC, Coleman TG (1967) Long-term regulation of the circulation: interrelationships with body fluid volumes. In: Physical bases of circulatory transport. Regulation and exchange. Philadelphia: WB Saunders

Guyton AC, Coleman TG (1969) Quantitative analysis of the pathophysiology of hypertension. Circ Res [Suppl 1:I-1] 24

Guyton AC, Coleman TG, Granger HJ (1972) Circulation: overall regulation. Annu Rev Physiol 34:13

Guyton AC, Coleman TG, Cowley AW Jr, Manning RD Jr, Norman RA Jr, Ferguson JD (1974) A systems analysis approach to understanding long-range arterial blood pressure control and hypertension. Circ Res 35:159

Guyton AC, Hall JE, Manning RD Jr, Norman RA Jr, DeClue JW (1978) A systems analysis of volume regulation. In Jorgensen CB, Shadhauge E (eds) Osmotic and volume regulation. Copenhagen: Munksgaard, p 283

Guyton AC (1980) Arterial pressure and hypertension. Philadelphia, WB Saunders (in press)

Hamilton WF, Richards DW (1964) The output of the heart. In: Fishman AP, Richards DW (eds) Circulation of the blood – men and ideas. New York: Oxford University Press, p 71

Heymans C, Bouckaert JJ (1934) Modifications de la pression arterielle après section des quatre nerfs frénateurs chez le chien. CR Soc Biol (Paris) 117:252

Koch E, Meis H (1929) Chronischer arterieller Hochdruck durch experimentelle Dauerausschaltung der Blutdruckzugler. Krankheitsforschung 7:241

Krogh A (1979) A supply of oxygen to the tissues and the regulation of the capillary circulation. J Physiol (Lond) 52:457

Langston JB, Guyton AC, Douglas BH, Dorsett PE (1963) Effect of changes in salt intake on arterial pressure and renal function in nephrectomized dogs. Circ Res 12:508

Ledingham JM, Cohen RD (1963) The role of the heart in the pathogenesis of renal hypertension. Lancet 2:979

Ledingham JM, Cohen RD (1964) Changes in extracellular fluid volume and cardiac output during the development of experimental renal hypertension. Can Med Assoc J 90:292

Manning RD Jr, Coleman TG, Guyton AC, Norman RA Jr, McCaa RE (1979) Essential role of mean circulatory filling pressure in salt-induced hypertension. Am J Physiol 236:R40

Page IH (1939) On the nature of the pressor action of renin. J Exp Med 70:521

Roy CS, Brown JG (1879) The blood pressure in variations in the arterioles, capillaries and smaller veins. J Physiol (Lond) 2:323

Rushmer RE, Smith DA Jr (1959) Cardiac control. Physiol Rev 39:11

Sarnoff SJ (1955) Myocardial contractility, as described by ventricular function curves: observations on Starling's law of the heart. Physiol Rev 35:107

Selkurt EE, Hall PW, Spencer MP (1949) Influence of graded arterial pressure decrement on renal clearance on creatinine, p-amino hippurate and sodium. Am J Physiol 159:369

Starling EH (1918) The Linacre Lecture on the Law of the Heart given at Cambridge, 1915. London: Longmans, Green

Sugimoto T, Sagawa K, Guyton AC (1966) Effect of tachycardia on cardiac output during normal and increased venous return. Am J Physiol 211:288

Traube L (1871) Über den Zusammenhang von Herz- und Nierenkrankheiten. Gesammelte Beiträge zur Pathologie und Physiologie, vol 2. Berlin: Hirschwald, p 290

HENRI DENOLIN

President of the European
Society of Cardiology

Closing remarks

This symposium was an unique opportunity to meet the famous pioneers of heart catheterization, of angiography, and of cardiac surgery. To hear them evaluating their experiences and to evaluate old and new methods was a real and great pleasure.

The development of cardiac catheterization and of angiography since 1940 was of tremendous importance as the beginning of a new era in cardiology, which changed completely the diagnostic and therapeutic approach of congenital and acquired heart disease. Even now, these methods remain essential in the evaluation of new noninvasive or less invasive methods of diagnosis. The future of the invasive methods remains difficult to evaluate today, but it is probably too early to announce the closure of the catheterization rooms, as was promised a few years ago by our colleagues involved in echocardiography. Further confrontation between invasive and noninvasive methods should be helpful for the definition of new attitudes, and the utilization of new diagnostic procedures.

In any case, a good knowledge of the work of the pioneers remains very useful: the technique of heart catheterization had already been described by Claude Bernard more than one hundred years ago, but was for a long time forgotten by the clinicians!

I hope that the Einthoven Foundation with the support of the European Society of Cardiology will help us to collect information on the history of our discipline. The educational value of the history of medicine, which is closely related to the general history of countries and of civilization, will be increased thereby. Also, a better understanding of the achievements in the past should be helpful to the research of our co-workers.

In the name of the participants of this symposium, I thank the organizers for giving us the opportunity to assist at a confrontation between the past, present and the future, and first of all Professor Snellen, who has always been so interested in the history of cardiology, being himself a member of a family in which medicine is an old tradition. I would like also to thank the dean of the Faculty, my friend Tammeling, and the co-organizer, Professor Arntzenius, as well as the other members of the Committee. We have of course to thank also the distinguished pioneers and famous scientists who accepted to be here, to recall the development of their work, to refresh our memories, and to enlighten the future.